Extra Treatises
Based on
Investigation & Inquiry

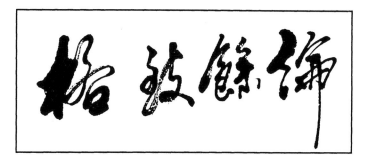

Extra Treatises
Based On
Investigation & Inquiry

A Translation of Zhu Dan-xi's
Ge Zhi Yu Lun

by Yang Shou-zhong & Duan Wu-jin

BLUE POPPY PRESS

Published by:

BLUE POPPY PRESS
A Division of Blue Poppy Enterprises, Inc.
3450 Penrose Place, Suite 110
BOULDER, CO 80301

First Edition April, 1994
Second Printing March, 1997
Third Printing August, 1998
Fourth Printing September, 1999

ISBN 0-936185-53-8

COMP Designation: Denotative translation

Printed at C & M Press, Denver, CO

10 9 8 7 6 5 4

Editor's Preface

This book is a translation of Zhu Dan-xi's *Ge Zhi Yu Lun (Extra Treatises Based on Investigation & Inquiry)*. Zhu Dan-xi, also known as Zhu Zhen-heng, was the founder of one of the four great schools of Chinese medicine during the Jin/Yuan dynasties. Best known for his statement, "Yang normally has a surplus, while yin is normally insufficient (*yang chang you yu, yin chang bu zu*)," the Reverend Dan Xi is remembered today as the progenitor of the School of Enriching Yin (*Zi Yin Pai*).

However, Zhu Dan-xi was the lineal recipient of the theories of all three other great masters of medicine during the Jin/Yuan dynasties. Rather than contending with or refuting the theories of Liu Wan-su, Zhang Zi-he, and Li Dong-yuan, Zhu extended and refined these. Zhu accepted Liu's beliefs that most disease is caused by or involves an element of evil heat. He also accepted Li's belief that this heat was frequently yin fire or damp heat. However, Zhu went on to explain the role of stirring ministerial fire in the production of internal heat. Although Zhu is remembered today for his insistence that yin is commonly insufficient, Zhu nonetheless used many of Li Dong-yuan's formulas and approaches to therapy based on supplementing and harmonizing the spleen and stomach. And although Zhu did not agree with Zhang Zi-he that all disease is due to the presence of evil qi, he was quite willing to use Zhang's methods of attack and precipitation with the proviso that the righteous qi not be injured by these harsh methods. Thus, in many respects, Zhu is not just one of four great masters but the culmination of Jin/Yuan medicine.

This book is a collection of medical essays written by Zhu. In each, he addresses some thorny issues in the practice of medicine during his time. In most of these, he first outlines a commonly held but overly simplistic belief regarding the disease or issue in question. Then he gives his own beliefs regarding the issue which he goes on to validate and defend by citing the *Nei Jing*, Zhang Zhong-jing, and other preeminent Chinese medical classics and great doctors of antiquity.

In particular, one of the recurrent themes of this book is Zhu's insistence that the practice of medicine must be more than the rote prescription of ancient or set formulas. He insists that the practice of medicine must be based on long learning and sound theory and that one should not rely on a simplistic, formulaic approach to prescription. In recounting his own apprenticeship under Luo Tai-wu, Zhu says, "During a year and a half, there was not (one) set formula (prescribed)." Zhu then goes on to quote a Master Xu, saying:

> I read (Zhang) Zhong-jing's book and use Zhong-jing's methodology, but I never confine (myself) to Zhong-jing's formulas. Only thus can I claim possession of Zhong-jing's heart.

Therefore, Zhu Dan-xi was one of the early, great proponents of individualized treatment based on a pattern diagnosis. This has today become the hallmark of the system of Chinese medicine which has come to be known in the West as Traditional Chinese Medicine or TCM.

This book also helps clarify the fact that TCM as a style of Chinese medicine is mostly a Confucian style. Although many Westerners think that TCM is based primarily on or somehow embodies the essence of Daoism, most of the great Chinese doctors of antiquity who advanced important new theories or wrote the classics of Chinese medicine were

Confucianists. This includes such great Chinese doctors as Zhang Zhong-jing, Huang-fu Mi, Li Dong-yuan, and Zhu Dan-xi. As the reader will see, Zhu very self-consciously and deliberately refers to himself as a Confucian and references the Confucian classics as his sources and models. More than once, his arguments revolve around the proper application of such Confucian principles as filial piety and the practice of compassion and moderation. As a *ru yi* or Confucian scholar doctor, Zhu Dan-xi is but one of the greatest of a long line of such scholar doctors who believed that the practice of medicine was a *dao* and a vehicle for enlightenment.

This book is a companion volume to Zhu Dan-xi's *Dan Xi Zhi Fa Xin Yao (The Heart & Essence of Dan Xi's Methods of Treatment)*. In that book, also translated by Yang Shou-zhong and published by Blue Poppy Press, Zhu primarily discusses the pattern differentiation treatment of a wide variety of internal and external diseases, whereas this book is primarily a book of theories and case histories exemplifying Zhu's application of those theories. Some terms translated in this book and some formulas appearing herein are explained more fully in notes to the *Xin Yao*. In addition, for more information about Zhu Dan-xi's life and place within the history of Chinese medicine, the reader is referred to Yang Shou-zhong's preface to *The Heart & Essence of Dan Xi's Methods of Treatment*. Readers interested in learning more about the Neoconfucian medicine of the Jin/Yuan dynasties and more about the teachings which influenced Zhu should see Li Dong-yuan's *Pi Wei Lun* published by Blue Poppy Press under the title, *Li Dong-yuan's Treatise on the Spleen & Stomach*.

As with other recent Blue Poppy Press publications, the translational terminology in this book is based on Nigel Wiseman's as given in his *Glossary of Chinese Medical Terms and Acupuncture Points*. Medicinal identifications are based on

Bensky & Gamble's *Chinese Herbal Medicine: Materia Medica*, Hong-yen Hsu's *Oriental Materia Medica: A Concise Guide*, and the Shanghai Science & Technology Press' *Zhong Yao Da Ci Dian (Encyclopedia of Chinese Medicinals)*. This translation is based on the 1985 Jiangsu Science and Technology Press edition edited by Mao Sun-tong.

Bob Flaws
October 19, 1993

Zhu Dan-xi's Preface

The *Su Wen (Simple Questions)* is a book conveying the *dao*. It is terse in wording and profound in meaning. (But) because it is farther and farther from the time (when it was composed, various) interpolations, errata, and deletions are not seldom encountered (when trying to read it). Thus it has become unreadable except by us (learned) Confucianists. Students hope to seek easy gains with comfort. (However,) when they see that this book is like a boundless ocean and reads as tastelessly as chewing wax, they abruptly declare that (such) ancient works are not appropriate for modern times. Bored, they forsake the book and, each following the other, begin to take to the study of the *Ju Fang (The Board's Formulary)*.[1] There are also numerous readers who intend to enhance their skills in the art (of healing) through reading but do so with a casual attitude and lack of perspicacity. It is this that is responsible for the obscurity and inscrutability of the medical *dao*! What a regret!

When I was 30 years old, my mother suffered from spleen pain, but the many attending physicians all threw up their hands in desperation. This struck in me a determination to learn medicine. Thereupon, I took up the *Su Wen* and began

---

[1]   The *Jiao Zheng Tai Ping Hui Min Ju Fang (Corrected & Collected Formulas of the Great Harmony Imperial Grace)* in full. This book, written between 1107—1110 CE by Chen Shi-wen and Pei Zhong-yuan, was a compendium of 297 formulas. By the time of Zhu Dan-xi, many doctors were prescribing from this book by rote in a symptomatic way with insufficient training in or understanding of Chinese medical theory and differential diagnosis.

to read it. In three years, I seemed to have some attainment. Two years later, my mother's illness was eased (*i.e.*, relieved) by (my) medication. I was (then) reminded of the internal damage of my late father, the cloudedness and oppression of the departed elder brother of my father, the nosebleeding of the departed younger brother of my father, the leg pain of my (own) young brother, and the accumulated phlegm of my wife. They all died from blunders in prescription. At this my heart and gallbladder broke with agony. There is no use repenting.

However, I was beset by worry that I was still partially in the dark concerning the study (of medicine). At the age of 40, I resumed reading the book (*i.e.*, the *Su Wen*). Because of my dull-wittedness, I ground myself in it day and night, leaving that which was doubtful and breaking through that which was understandable.

Another four years passed, and I came across the privilege of being instructed by Master Luo, the Great Void, name taboo Zhi Di, and therefore had access to the works of (Liu) He-jian[2], (Zhang) Dai-ren[3], (Li) Dong-yuan[4], and (Wang) Hai-

---

[2]   Liu He-jian, a.k.a. Liu Shou-zhen, a.k.a. Liu Wan-su, circa 1120-1200 CE. Liu was the founder of the *Han Liang Pai* or School of Cold and Cool (Medicine). He believed that most pathologies involved heat and, therefore, should be treated primarily by clearing heat with bitter, cold medicinals.

[3]   Zhang Dai-ren, a.k.a. Zhang Cong-zheng, a.k.a. Zhang Zi-he, circa 1156—1228 CE. Zhang was the founder of the *Gong Xia Pai* or School of Attack & Precipitation (*i.e.*, Purgation). He believed that all disease was due to the presence of some evil qi. Therefore, he believed that the main methods of treatment were those that rid the presence of evil qi from the body. His three methods consisted of precipitation, emesis, and diaphoresis.

cang[5]. Only then did I realize that damp heat and ministerial fire are the common causes of disease. (With this, I) came to the recognition that, in regard to medical books, a sound theory cannot be established without the *Su Wen*, and further that nothing short of the *Ben Cao (Materia Medica)*[6] can provide a rule for (composing) formulas.

How can one identify disease if one possesses formulas but has no theory? (Whereas,) equipped with theory but possessing no formulas, how can one (design them by) copying (others')? The books of (Zhang) Zhong-jing[7] provide de-

---

[4] Li Dong-yuan, a.k.a. Li Gao, 1180—1251 CE, author of the *Pi Wei Lun (Treatise on the Spleen & Stomach)*. Li was the founder of the *Bu Tu Pai* or School of Supplementing Yin. Besides emphasizing the role of the spleen and stomach in diseases involving counterflow inversion, Li also refined Liu He-jian's ideas about yin fire, *i.e.*, damp heat, being the most common cause of disease.

[5] A.k.a. Wang Hao-gu, pupil to Zhang Yuan-su and Li Gao, a prolific author of medical works.

[6] *I.e.*, the *Shen Nong Ben Cao Jing (Shen Nong's Materia Medica Classic)* in full, the first Chinese materia medica believed to have been written in the Han dynasty. This book was later re-edited by Tao Hong-jing, 456—536 CE. This book is also referred to as the *Ben Cao Jing (Materia Medica Classic)* or even more simply as the *Ben Jing*.

[7] Zhang Zhong-jing, 142—220 CE, author of the *Shang Han Lun (Treatise on Damage by Cold)* and the *Jin Gui Yao Lue (Prescriptions from the Golden Cabinet)*. These are the first Chinese books on the application of the *bian zheng lun zhi* methodology to the prescription of herbal formulas. *Bian zheng lun zhi* refers to the basing of treatment on a discrimination of patterns. Zhang outlined six stages (*liu fen*) in the progression of cold damage from the outside to the inside with differential signs and symptoms and separate formulas for each stage. These formulas are, to this day, referred to as *jing fang*, classical

tailed discussions of external contraction with their theories elaborated in the form of question and answer; while the books of (Li) Dong-yuan, with their explicit explanations on the natures and flavors (of medicinals), give detailed account of internal damage. It is only with these books that medicine begins to be comprehensive, and, as a *dao*, it is only with these that medicine begins to be enlightening. Therefore, I cannot help being skeptical of the *Ju Fang*. That book has been current since the Song dynasty, spreading far and wide in the south and north, and gradually becoming popular with the people. (And) there is certainly some reason for its popularity. (However,) this situation has caused me to look long (at the fact that the theory of) damp heat and ministerial fire has been retreating into oblivion since Supreme Servant (Wang)[8] who supplied annotations (to the *Su Wen*). And it was not till (my) various predecessors, like Zhang (Dai-ren) and (Li) Dong-yuan, that (this theory) has begun to be illuminated.

In the human body, yin is (commonly) insufficient and yang is superabundant. This statement is clearly reiterated in the *Su Wen*, but many of our predecessors have never advanced it, thus facilitating the flourishing of the *Ju Fang*. In spite of my rudimentary and partial learning, I have ventured to give

---

formulas or as *gu fang*, ancient formulas. Zhang Zhong-jing's books are the *locus classicus* of the Chinese herbal formulary literature in the same way that the *Shen Nong Ben Cao Jing* is the *locus classicus* of the Chinese materia medica literature.

8   Wang Tai-pu, a.k.a. Wang Bing (710—804 CE). *Tai Pu* means Supreme Servant and is the name of an imperial office. The Supreme Servant was a post in charge of carriages, hunting, and livestock of the royal family and the dressing of the emperor in particular. Wang Bing was the first person to completely edit, collate, (and some people say, add chapters to) the *Nei Jing*.

an explanation concerning part of the *Su Wen* and, in addition, illustrations concerning the treatment methods of the *Jin Gui (Golden Cabinet)*.[9] (I have done this) in order to give evidence of the defects of the *Ju Fang* and, occasionally, to supplement my own ideas in the back (of this book).

The ancients regarded medicine as a body of knowledge derived from investigation and enquiry by us Confucianists. Therefore, (I) have titled this book *Extra Treatises Based on Investigation and Inquiry*. It remains, however, (for future generations) to ascertain whether the result of my efforts is positive. I sincerely hope that gentlemen[10] will make corrections in the years to come.

---

[9] *I.e.*, the *Jin Gui Yao Lue (Prescriptions from the Golden Cabinet)* in full. This is the companion volume to Zhang Zhong-jing's *Shang Han Lun (Treatise on Damage by Cold)* written in the late Han dynasty. While the later book primarily deals with the treatment of exogenous disease, the former book primarily describes the treatment of endogenous diseases, gynecological diseases, pediatric diseases, and diseases due to faulty diet.

[10] *I.e.*, men of moral character, as defined by Confucianism.

Table of Contents

Table of Contents

Table of Contents

Table of Contents

Prologue to Admonitions on Food & Drink and Sexual Desire

It is stated in the *Zhuan (Commentaries)*[1] that human beings' great desires are for food and drink and sex. I often think to myself that desire for sex does (in fact) matter greatly and that the desire for food and drink concerns the body particularly closely. In the world, there are not a few who, one after another, become sunk deeply into such desires. If anyone really intends to devote themself to the *dao*, they must first take the study of this (problem) to heart. Therefore, I shall (begin by) making two admonitions, (one) concerning the desire for food and drink and (the other) concerning sexual desire. (These) are intended for my relatives of the younger generation as well as my comrades.

---

[1]   *I.e.*, the *Yi Zhuan (The Exposition of the [Classic of] Change)* of which there are different versions.

1

Admonitions on Food & Drink

The human body is precious (because) it is inherited from one's parents.[2] Yet there are no end of cases where the body is damaged for the sake of the mouth. Because a person has a body, hunger and thirst arise repeatedly, and subsequently (one) does have to eat and drink in order to continue their life. (However,) one can see that, in the muddle-headed, it is because of indulgence in good tastes which leads to excess of the five flavors that diseases spring up in swarms.

(In the beginning,) the generation of an illness presents with a very fine mechanism, (merely) the sudden disappearance of desire for that which (previously) drew out gluttonous drool from the mouth. When the disease is fully developed, both food and drink are forsaken! (Then) the parents are left with worry and the physicians must pray (*i. e.*, resort) to a hundred (medical) stratagems. Those poor and humble in the mountains and wilderness know nothing but bland and homely (diet), but their movements never betray decrepitude and their bodies remain safe and sound (their entire lives). Qi is evenly shared (among all people), and their bodies are the same. Therefore, why am I alone taken with many diseases? If repentance and enlightenment are germinated, (one will be) like a mirror becoming clear once the dust (is wiped off) and will keep an abstemious diet forever.

---

[2]   According to Confucian doctrine, the body is inherited from the parents or ancestors and must be returned intact to the ancestors upon death. While living, care of the body, which, in a sense, does not belong to the individual alone, is part of one's filial piety or obligation to one's family.

(As it is said) in the "*Xiang Ci* (Caption of the Diagrams)" in the *Yi ([Classic of] Change)*[3], "The small may be nursed to result in a great loss." Or, as Mencius has mocked, "The mouth is capable of causing disease and also of ruining one's virtue." Keep the mouth (shut) like a (sealed) bottle, and persevere in practicing this without boredom or relaxation.

Admonitions on Sexual Desire

Human life corresponds with heaven and earth. The *kun* (*i.e.*, earthly) *dao* becomes women, (while) the *qian* (*i.e.*, heavenly) *dao* becomes men. These are wedded as husband and wife and reproduction relies on them. This demands good timing, (*i.e.*,) a time when the blood and qi are upright and strong. Love-making should be carried out with civility, and intercourse should occur at intervals (*i.e.*, at opportune times). These are essential if there is to be affinity between father and son. It is observed that those muddle-headed (ones who) submit to their passions and resign themselves to (sexual) desire, with only the fear that their excessive (desire) cannot be satisfied, (thus cause) an abundance of dry toxins[4] (to be generated in their bodies).

---

3   This refers to the *Yi Jing (Classic of Change)*. It is believed that the commentaries on the 64 hexagrams were written by King Wen of the Zhou dynasty circa 1143 BCE. Therefore, this preeminent Chinese classic is also referred to as the *Zhou Yi*.

4   Because essence is yin, emission or ejaculation of reproductive essence is believed to consume yin. Since yin is associated with moisture and wetness, such consumption of yin then leads to dry toxins.

Qi (which is) yang and blood (which is) yin are the spirit of the human body. If yin is quiet and yang is sound, our bodies (enjoy) a long (*i.e.*, lasting) spring. How little blood and qi are there (in the body) and how can we not be frugal of them? The offspring born by us may turn into the robber of our blood and qi! If a woman gives herself up, her sexual desire may be really excessive. (But) a strict bedroom is the guarantee of a harmonious house. If a man gives himself up, his family is ruined. Not only is he forsaking virtue, but his body is wasted. Keep away from the bed-curtains and the libidinous heart will be withdrawn. (Then) food and drink will become sweet and delicious, the body will become fit, and disease will heal.

Treatise on Yang Being Superabundant and Yin Being Insufficient

Humans receive qi from heaven and earth and thus there is life. The yang qi of heaven becomes qi, while the yin qi of the earth becomes blood. Therefore, qi normally has a surplus, while blood normally is insufficient. What is the justification for saying this?

Heaven and earth are the parents of the ten of thousand things. Great is heaven which is yang, moving around the earth. While earth, lying in the center of heaven, is yin and is held up by the great qi of heaven. The sun, solid, is also yang. It moves outside the moon, while the moon, (capable) of waning, is yin. It is bright by dint of the sun's light. The

4

yin qi in the human body ebbs and flows depending on the waxing and waning of the moon. As far as human life is concerned, a male begins to have free flow of essence at the age of 16, while a female's (menstrual) flow (begins at) 14. After being given shape, (the body) still is built by breast milk and water and grains for nourishment. When yin qi is (fully) developed, it is able to copulate with yang qi. Therefore, people cannot become parents until they are grown (and their yin is mature).

Ancient people did not marry until near to the age of 30 or (at least) after 20. This shows how difficult it is for yin qi to develop and how good the ancient people were at containing and nurturing themselves. A note in the *Li Ji (Records of Rites)*[5] says, "Only those that give (particular attention to) nurturing yin after 50 years of age can enjoy accretion (of life span)." The *Nei Jing (Inner Classic)* states, "At the age of 40 yin qi is automatically reduced by half, and one's daily life activities become debilitated." It adds, "In males, the essence runs out at the age of 64, while in females menstruation ceases at the age of 49." After (its full) development, yin qi provides supplies for no more than 30 years for vision, hearing, speech, and movement, and by then has become depleted. (However,) human beings' sexual desire can be boundless. How can yin qi, which is hard to develop but easy to deplete, provide supplies (to meet the demands of) such desire?

It is stated in the classic (*i.e.*, the *Nei Jing*), "Yang is the heavenly qi, governing the external, and yin is the earthly qi, governing the internal." Therefore, the yang tract is replete,

---

[5]   This is one of the five Confucian classics, the other four being the *Shi (Poetry)*, *Shu (History)*, *Yi ([Classic of] Change)*, and the *Chun Qiu (Spring & Autumn [Annals])*.

while the yin tract is vacuous. It is also said, "If consummate yin is vacuous, heavenly qi expires, (but if) consummate yang is exuberant, earthly qi is insufficient." Thus this view concerning the whereabouts of vacuity and exuberance is not (some) far-fetched argument of mine.

The kidneys govern blocking and storage, and the liver manages coursing and draining. Both of these viscera are possessed of ministerial fire whose ligation homes to the heart above. The heart is sovereign fire and easily becomes stirred when affected by things. Once the heart stirs, ministerial fire stirs too. When ministerial fire stirs, essence escapes on its own. (Thus) when ministerial fire arises vehemently, (essence) flows in the dark, discharged and drained even not during coitus. That is why the sages always instruct people to withdraw and nourish the heart. Their meaning is profound.

Heaven and earth produce the four seasons by means of change (*i.e.,*) the debility and effulgence of the five phases. The five viscera and the six bowels of humans also undergo debility and effulgence in response. The fourth month which is ascribed to *si* (B6) and the fifth month which is ascribed to *wu* (B7) are (the months when) fire is greatly effulgent. Fire is the husband[6] of lung metal. When it is effulgent, metal is debilitated. The sixth month which is ascribed to *wei* (B8) is (a month when) earth is greatly effulgent. Earth is the husband of water, and when it is effulgent, water is debilitated. Moreover, kidney water must constantly rely on lung metal as its mother to supplement and help its deficiency.

For these reasons, the *Nei Jing* repeatedly instructs to enrich

---

6   In ancient China, the husband lorded over the wife. Therefore, this refers to the restraining or controlling phase.

the source of transformation. In summer, ancient people preferred, as a rule, to sleep alone and have bland flavored (food, thus) cautiously and conscientiously taking care (of the source). The two viscera of metal and water should be protected and nurtured because of nothing other than their detestation for effulgent fire and earth. The *Nei Jing* states, "Those who do not store essence in winter will invariably contract warm disease in spring." The tenth month which is ascribed to *hai* (B12) and the eleventh month which is ascribed to *zi* (B1) are the very (times) when fire and qi are lying deep, shut in and stored so as to nourish the true of the root. This is the root which generates and upstirs in the coming spring. If it is mutilated and plundered by self-indulgence in taste and (sexual) desire at this time (*i.e.*, winter), there will be no root below at the time when spring is upraising. (Thus) yang qi becomes buoyant and floating, and warm and hot diseases will invariably arise.

Fire and earth being effulgent in the summer months and fire and qi lying deep in the winter months are spoken of as the vacuity of the year. Prior to the first quarter, the moon is but an outline, and after the last quarter, the moon is empty. This is also a vacuity, (a vacuity) of the month. Great wind, great fog, rainbows and lightening, sudden cold and sudden heat, solar and lunar eclipses, worry and anxiety, wrath and anger, fear and fright, sorrow and melancholy, intoxication and overeating, taxation and fatigue, preoccupation and toil are also all vacuities, (*i.e.*, vacuities) of the day. (Further) when a disease or affliction is beginning to abate or sores are just breaking out, there is vacuity of more than one day. Nowadays, between the end of spring and the beginning of summer, many (people) suffer from headache, weak feet, reduced food intake, and body heat. This is the illness described by (Zhang) Zhong-jing as exacerbated during spring and summer but relieved in autumn and winter. (Its) pulse is wiry and large. It is also popularly known as summer sickness.[7] If one commits the offenses of those four kinds of vacuity[8], it is difficult to escape from this disease.

Whenever it is mentioned that senile looks appear just at a robust age with everything spoiled in terms of both supporting (one's) elders and looking after (one's) young, one cannot help being deeply struck by fright and shock. The ancients said, "See not that which is desired, and the heart will be kept from being upset." If gentleness and softness overwhelm the body, (if lovely) sound and voice overwhelm the ears, (if attractive) colors overwhelm the eyes, and (if) aromatic and sweet smells overwhelm the nose, who is (such) an iron person whose heart can remain unmoved? Those who are good at containing life live away from their home during the (above said) five months. (And) when it is the vacuity of the month, it is proper to keep away from the bed-curtains. (The husband and wife) should both pay their respects to (their bodies and thus to their ancestors) and protect and keep wholesome the celestial harmony. (I) wish (the reader) not to violate these teachings concerning paying respect to the body. This is (my) great hope.

---

[7]   This refers to a type of disease due to vacuity and weakness of spleen and stomach or to insufficiency of yin qi. It is so named because it always occurs in the summer months as a seasonal disease.

[8]   The four kinds of vacuity are vacuity of the year, month, and day, and the vacuity of more than one day, *i.e.*, a disease beginning to abate or sores just breaking out.

Treatise on the Necessity of Tracing the Root in the Treatment of Disease

(Just) as grass has its roots, so disease has its root. If one cuts off the leaves without eradicating the root, the grass will still stand there. Treating disease is like weeding. Treating a bowel when the disease is in the viscus or attacking the interior when the disease is in the exterior can not only mutilate and plunder the stomach qi but also enrich and assist the disease evil. How can (such) a physician be called a physician?

A clan grandfather of mine, aged 70, with a strong physique but a very thin form, suffered from diarrhea late in the summer. This persisted till deep in the autumn and responded to none of a hundred formulas. On the day I saw him, although his disease had lasted long, his spirit was not withered. (He) had inhibited voiding of scant urine which, however, was not dark-colored and his pulse at both hands was choppy and rather wiry. He himself said that he felt a little oppression at the diaphragm and, in addition, food intake was reduced. From this I realized (his situation). I said that there must be years long, deep accumulation tucked in (his) stomach and intestines. When asked what his favorite food in life was, he replied, "I like to eat carp best of all, and I have never been short of it for one day in the past three years." (Hearing this,) I said that there was accumulated phlegm in (his) lungs.

Because the lungs are the viscera of the large intestine, the (problem) ought to be that the root of the large intestine was insecure. It was necessary to clarify the source, and then the flow would naturally become clear. (He was then bid to) take Fructus Evodiae Rutecarpae (*Zhu Yu*), Pericarpium Citri Reticulatae (*Chen Pi*), fresh Herba Allii Fistulosi (*Qing Cong*), Radix Medicagonis Sativae (*Xu Mu Gen*), and raw Rhizoma Zingiberis (*Sheng Jiang*). These were boiled down into a thick decoction of about one bowlful and drunk with granulated sugar. Then (he was instructed) to probe the throat with his own fingers. Half a watch later, about one half *sheng* of phlegm was vomited which was (sticky) like glue. That very night (his condition) reduced by half. The next morning he again drank (the formula) and again vomited one half *sheng* of phlegm. (Then) the diarrhea stopped. After that (he) was administered *Ping Wei San* (Level the Stomach Powder) with Rhizoma Atractylodis Macrocephalae (*Bai Zhu*) and Rhizoma Coptidis Chinensis (*Huang Lian*) added. Ten days later (he) was at ease.

Wang Zhong-yan of Dong Yang[9] came across me on the way, asking me, "Every day when I eat, the food must go across the diaphragm in a winding way. Moreover, it feels hard and rough, giving a little pain. Except for this, I have no (other) afflictions. What kind of disease is this?" His pulse felt very choppy on the right (hand), particularly deep in the *guan* section, but harmonious on the left (hand). I answered "Static blood exists in the opening of the stomach venter. Because of depression, qi has formed into phlegm. This must have been caused by (a certain kind of) food. Tell me plainly what (kind of food) it is." He could not think of it either. I went on, "What kind of substance did you take most of all in the previous winter?" He answered, "Every day I used to drink two or three cups of wine to force out the cold qi in

---

9   Dong Yang is a county in Zhejiang province today.

the morning." (Therefore, I) designed for him a formula (which consisted of) drinking one half silver cup of cold Succus Allii Tuberosi (*Jiu Zhi*) sip by sip (every day). When one half *jin* of chive juice was thus consumed, his disease would be overcome. Later (my words) proved true.

Again, in early summer, a next-door neighbor of mine, aged over 30, contracted loose bowels with a little oppression above the diaphragm. He was crafty and irritable by nature and had been suffering from lower body *gan* sore which had been relieved but now had relapsed. A physician administered him two doses of *Zhi Zhong Tang* (Treat the Center Decoction)[10], and (subsequently) he was taken with cloudedness and oppression as if dying. After a little while, (he) resurrected. I palpated his pulse which was choppy on both hands, a bit wiry, and somewhat rapid at the deep level. I concluded that this was a severe and recalcitrant case of lower body *gan* sore and prescribed *Dang Gui Long Hui Wan* (*Dang Gui*, Gentiana & Aloe Pills) with Secretio Moschi Moschiferi (*She Xiang*) removed. Four doses (administered) and (his) loose bowels were improved. Then (I) administered *Xiao Chai Hu* (Minor Bupleurum [Decoction]) with Rhizoma Pinelliae Ternatae (*Ban Xia*) removed and Rhizoma Coptidis Chinensis (*Huang Lian*), Radix Paeoniae Lactiflorae (*Shao Yao*), Rhizoma Ligustici Wallichii (*Chuan Xiong*), and fresh Rhizoma Zingiberis (*Sheng Jiang*) added. (All these) were boiled. (After) five or six doses (were administered), recovery ensued.

These three persons all had choppy pulses, wiry or not wiry,

---

10 This is composed of Radix Panacis Ginseng (*Ren Shen*), blast-fried Rhizoma Zingiberis (*Pao Jiang*), Rhizoma Atractylodis Macrocephalae (*Bai Zhu*), Radix Glycyrrhizae (*Gan Cao*), Pericarpium Citri Reticulatae (*Chen Pi*), and Pericarpium Viridis Citri Reticulatae (*Qing Pi*).

but the treatment methods were different (in each case). How (else) can one work out (their proper) medication, if not by tracing the roots (of their disease)?

Treatise on the Choppy Pulse

In humans, for (every) one exhalation, the pulse moves three *cun*. Likewise, for (every) one inhalation, it moves (another) three *cun*. (Thus) for one whole respiration, the pulse moves six *cun*. During a day and night, there are 13,500 respirations and (therefore) the pulse moves 810 *zhang*.[11] These numbers are constants in the circulation of blood and qi in normal people.

If a physician intends to determine whether the blood and qi are diseased or not, they have no other way to obtain that knowledge than by palpating the pulse. The pulse can present a number of different images, and the types that are recorded in the *Mai Jing (Pulse Classic)*[12] are twenty plus four (in number), namely, the floating, deep, scallion-stalk, slippery, replete, wiry, tight, surging, faint, moderate or relaxed, choppy, slow, hidden, soggy, weak, rapid, thin, stirring, vacuous, skipping, bound, regularly interrupted,

---

[11] One *zhang* equals 3.3 meters

[12] This is the earliest and most comprehensive book extant on the pulse. It was written by Wang Shu-he in the third century CE. It was then translated into many languages, including Arabic. Many of its insights were incorporated into Tibetan, Mongolian, Unani, Ayurvedic, and Western scholastic medicines.

drumskin, and scattered (pulses). Usually (more than one of) these images are seen in combination.

The diseases in human beings fall into four (categories), known as cold, heat, repletion, and vacuity. Therefore, the student of the pulse should take the floating, sinking, slow, and rapid (pulses) as the reins in observing disease conditions. This is a unchanging principle. It is true that the appearance of a choppy (pulse) indicates mostly vacuity and cold, but, in some cases, intractable heat is the cause of a disease with a vacuous pulse. Whenever physicians find a (pulse) image of insufficient qi under their fingers, if they consider it as vacuity or cold and imprudently prescribe medicinals which are nothing short of hot supplementing ones, there will be many cases of moderate ailments becoming severe and severe diseases ending in death.

Why is this? That which humans depend on for life is blood and qi. Either because of melancholy or thick flavors, absence of sweating or supplementing formulas, qi may soar up and blood boil. The clear will (thus) transform into the turbid, and old phlegm and retained rheum will congeal, become sticky, mix together, and coagulate. (In that case, since) the pulse passageways are obstructed and inhibited, they are no longer able to circulate by themselves. (Thus they) also display a choppy image. If the pulse appears somewhat strong and rapid as well when felt at the bone level with heavy pressure applied, (one) should appeal to reflection and examine the signs. A diagnosis of intractable heat is justified only there is a heat pattern in terms of form and qi. This is an instruction intended for beginners and will certainly be considered superfluous by learned and experienced scholars.

A Master Wu of Dong Yang was only 50 years of age, had a fat form, and used to have thick flavored (food). Moreover,

13

he was subject to depression and irritability and often (his) pulse was deep and choppy. Since the beginning of spring, he had contracted a disease of phlegm qi. The (attending) physician thought it was vacuity cold and administered entirely dry, hot, aromatic, and penetrating medicinals. During the fourth month, his feet became weak with qi upsurging and food intake reduced. I was sent for a treatment. I said that this was heat depression with a vacuous spleen giving rise to a pattern of atonic inversion. A fat form with a deep pulse indicated no mortal pattern, but (now) the medicinal evils were too exuberant. At this juncture of effulgent fire, there was really hardly any hope of survival. (Although I was aware of little I could do), I prescribed as a stopgap measure a paste made from Rhizoma Atractylodis Macrocephalae (*Bai Zhu*) taken with Succus Bambusae (*Zhu Li*). When 2 *jin* (of Atractylodes) was (thus) consumed, qi was borne down and food intake increased. One month later, (however,) a massive sweating was followed by death. This is written as a lesson in order for the wise not to take the same disastrous road.

Treatise on Nurturing the Aged

After people live to (their) 60s or 70s, both their essence and blood are consumed. Even though their life is normal and not (particularly) eventful, they may present heat signs. What (are these signs)? Clouded head, gum in the eyes, itchy muscles, frequent voiding of urine, (spontaneous discharge of) nasal mucus, teeth loss, copious drooling, little sleep, weak feet, dull ears, impaired memory, dizziness, dry intestines (*i.e.*, dry stools), a grimy facial complexion, hair

14

loss, flowery vision, long sitting and dozing off, cold without exposure to wind, hungering soon after eating, and tearing when laughing. Anyone who has entered the aged state cannot but have such signs.

It may be argued, "It is appropriate to administer old people in great amounts elixirs (made from) *Wu* (Radix Aconiti) and *Fu* (Radix Praeparatus Aconiti Carmichaeli) in the *Ju Fang*. Is this not reasonable (since) their qi is weak with age but not yet vacuous and does this not well justify warm supplementation? (But) now your honor thinks all those signs to be of heat. (Therefore, does this not mean) that these elixirs should not be applied in old people?" My answer is that not only the elixirs from Radix Aconiti and Radix Praeparatus Aconiti Carmichaeli cannot be used unwarrantedly, but good wine and fat meat, sodden wheat-flour foods and oil, roasted, stewed, and fried (foods), and acrid, pungent, sweet, and greasy (foods) are all included among the prohibited.

Some may exclaim, "How stupid you are! Sweetness and fat nourish the aged, and there are instructions in the classics that bear this out. If a son or a daughter-in-law provides (their parents) with inadequate supplies of sweetness and fat, they are showing a lack of filial piety. Now suppose what you say were true, what theory do you have that can justify this (ethically)? We would like to hear it in a few words." To this I would respond, sorrowfully, by saying, "The very saying applies here that the *dao* can carry on parallel and without contradiction." Now allow me to explain this in detail. In ancient times, there was the Nine Squares system of land ownership,[13] and neighborhood and village school-

---

13 This refers to a system of land ownership in ancient China. It consisted of one large square field divided into nine smaller ones like

ing was prosperous. Everyone knew how to behave themselves civilly and courteously, and each household was worthy of being dubbed a title. Meat was unaccessible to either the young or the middle-aged, and (people) did not have meat until 50 years old. (Nowadays, however, people) are greedy and gluttonous while they are strong and robust, and, by 50, illnesses have already broken out in them in great number with (their) qi consumed and blood exhausted, sinews flaccid and bones atonic, (their) stomach and intestines congested and stagnated, and drool and foam brimming over. In addition, yin in the human body is difficult to develop but easy to deplete. After 60 or 70 years of age, yin becomes too insufficient to match yang. Whereas solitary yang is all but on the verge of flying away, soaring up. It is only because the prenatal stomach qi still, for the time being, lingers and also due to the strength of yin from water and grains that solitary yang, confined by these bonds, yet stays put.

These are all (signs) of scant blood. The *Nei Jing* states, "The kidneys are averse to dryness." (Yet) what are elixirs (made) from Radix Aconiti and Radix Praeparatus Aconiti Carmichaeli if not dry? For people with scant blood, such medicinals as Radix Ledebouriellae Sesloidis (*Fang Feng*), Rhizoma Pinelliae Ternatae (*Ban Xia*), Rhizoma Atractylodis (*Cang Zhu*), and Rhizoma Cyperi Rotundi (*Xiang Fu*), as long as they are dry medicinals, dare not be administered in large quantities, let alone elixirs (made) from Radix Aconiti and Radix Praeparatus Aconiti Carmichaeli.

---

the Chinese character *jing* (井) meaning a well or spring. Each peripheral plot was owned by a different household, while the central one was owned by all.

One may continue to argue, "Since the whole *Ju Fang* prescribes nothing but warm and hot (medicinals) to nurture yang, are not your honor's words fallacious and absurd?" My response is that when the *Ju Fang* prescribes dry formulas, it aims at thwarting damp disease. Once dampness obtains dryness, it is surely remitted. When the *Ju Fang* prescribes warm formulas, it aims at thwarting vacuity disease.

(However,) it is better to supplement the spleen than the kidneys. When helped by warmth, the spleen is enabled to transform easily, and taste of food (*i.e.*, the appetite) increases. Even though there is still vacuity below temporarily, (the whole condition) may improve after a little while. The *Nei Jing's* treatment method also implies the use of thwarting. This (method) has been presumably devised for those of thick constitution with shallow(-rooted) disease. This (method) is also used by Confucian scholar (physicians) as a stopgap (measure. However,) if (this method) is used constantly (*i.e.*, routinely), is not that a gross blunder?

In those who are aged, their constitution, thick as it may have been, is now nearly too thin. (Although their) disease may be shallow, their root is easy to pull out. (Then) how can thwarting medicinals be employed to achieve a rapid effect? Those of fat form with scant blood and those of thin form with replete qi may occasionally be treated with thwarting medicinals. (Yet even in these cases,) if (the condition) gets out of hand, what can one take as a remedy? I would rather take a little time beforehand to think of a perfectly safe plan (of action). Is not this nice (*i.e.*, preferable)? The reason should now be clear why elixirs (made) from Radix Aconiti and Radix Praeparatus Aconiti Carmichaeli should not be administered recklessly.

As for food and drink, it is especially necessary to remain

abstemious (in one's diet). Old people have internal vacuity with a weak spleen and yin depletion with a quick temper. Internal vacuity and a hot stomach result in rapid hungering with desire for food, while eating (but little) with a weak spleen which transforms (food) with difficulty leads to surfeit. When yin is vacuous, it is difficult (for qi) to descend. Consequently qi is depressed into phlegm. As for vision, hearing, speech, and movement, all of these are disabled (or) sluggish. (Old people) are discontented in a hundred ways, and the fire of (their) anger easily burns. Even though their sons are filial and grandsons docile, they tend to stamp the floor with anger over the (merest) trifle. (And) what if their sons and grandsons are not filial and obedient? Therefore, it is clear why foods (which are) hot in nature, are prepared (directly) over a charcoal fire, are fragrant and pungent in qi, or are sweet and oily in flavor are all unfit (for the old) to take.

According to popular opinion, those who have a sturdy, thick stomach and intestines and who have a stupendous fortune may as well enjoy rich supplies of nourishment. (But) being resigned to the mouth is really a treat (only) for a moment. Accumulation will, over time, certainly result in disaster. From this point of view, the less (such treats), the better, and none is best (of all). To please the mouth causes disease and thick flavored (food) contains toxins. This maxim of past sages still rings true in our ears. How can one not be prudent?

Again some might ask, "(Suppose we believe) what you have said is true. Could you feel at ease if you denied (delicious food) to one who is bordering on expiry?" (To those) I would say that a gentleman loves people by way of virtue, while a base person does so by way of appeasement. What if one is treating one's respected (elders)? Food and drink are (provided) in order to nurture life, not to cause disease. If that which (is meant) to nurture turns out to be that which brings damage, (I am) afraid it is not what a gentleman means by piety and respect.

"If that is so, what kind of behavior is proper?" The answer is that to love life and hate death, to love fitness and to hate disease are common emotions among human beings. As a son or a grandson, one should first reason with sincerity and convincing words (with the elder on) the whys and wherefores (of their diet. They should) explain the natures of substances, make use of analogy and metaphor, and count up the gains and losses. All this should be done respectfully and cautiously. Secondly, one should set an example (themself. Thus the elder) will certainly be moved and enlightened while (at the same time) one is free from the misdemeanor of opposition and antagonism.

Your honor just mentioned denial to those (about to) expire. This (teaching involves) more than a (single) act of filial piety applied to the sick. When healthy, (the elder) may be supplied with a certain substance on a regular basis after careful consideration of its appropriateness. If (the elder) will not take a food, substitute another. How can this mar (one's) filial piety? If, when life is uneventful, one keeps (their) mouth shut (to their elder), never uttering a word of exhortation or persuasion to straighten things out, how then can one prohibit (the sick elder from taking some inappropriately desired food and drink) once (their) hungry intestines are rumbling with gluttonous drool already running and with the food and drink in front sending a fragrant, sweet smell straight into (their) nose? The classics instruct that one should feed (their elders) with a sense of loyalty. (I think) the implication of the word loyalty agrees with this meaning. Please do not overlook this (problem) too easily.

19

Although compared with the ancients I feel ashamed for my attendance upon my old mother, when over 70, she did not have fits of copious phlegm and rheum which she had suffered from before. (I) assume (from this fact) that (I finally) had obtained the *dao* of abstemious nurturing and had learned the art (of attending to the old). Once, because she had dry bound stools, I prepared her well-done gruel mixed with fresh cow's milk and pig's fat. Although this achieved temporary lubrication and disinhibition, slimy substance eventually accumulated in great quantities. The next summer it became depressed into sticky phlegm, giving rise to lateral costal sores. She suffered from this affliction for days on end. (She was) upset and despondent (whether) awake or asleep. As her son, I could find no place to hide (my) shame. Therefore, I reflected painstakingly and (eventually) harvested with the idea of abstemious nurturing. I regularly administered her such stomach and blood-supplementing medicinals as Radix Panacis Ginseng (*Ren Shen*) and Rhizoma Atractylodis Macrocephalae (*Bai Zhu*) and made some modification (to the formula) in accordance with the seasons. As a result, her stools were no longer dry, (and she had) a bright, shining facial complexion. Although she looked emaciated and weak, she had no disease at all. She enjoyed a peaceful life in her old age all thanks to this.

Thus (I) designed a formula which consists of Radix Panacis Ginseng (*Ren Shen*) and Rhizoma Atractylodis Macrocephalae (*Bai Zhu*) as the sovereigns, Radix Achyranthis Bidentatae (*Niu Xi*) and Radix Paeoniae Lactiflorae (*Shao Yao*) as the ministers, and Pericarpium Citri Reticulatae (*Chen Pi*) and Sclerotium Poriae Cocos (*Fu Ling*) as the assistants. In spring, add Rhizoma Ligustici Wallichii (*Chuan Xiong*). In summer, add Fructus Schizandrae Chinensis (*Wu Wei Zi*), Radix Scutellariae Baicalensis (*Huang Qin*), and Tuber Ophiopogonis Japonicae (*Mai Men Dong.* And) in winter, add Radix Angelicae Sinensis (*Dang Gui Shen*) and double the amount of fresh Rhizoma Zingiberis (*Sheng Jiang*. Give) one or two doses a day. Administer this formula immediately once short voiding of scant urine is heard. Restoration of urination to normal duration is a short cut in eliminating disease (from old persons).

Later in Dong Yang, I heard of an old Serene Lady[14] named He who was smart and intelligent. From 70 years old onward, whenever she felt a little unwell, she would give up gruel for days and have merely several doses of a decoction of Radix Panacis Ginseng (*Ren Shen*. With this, her condition) would stop. Eventually she lived to over ninety years old and died a death from no disease. Her case chances to agree (with my views stated above), so I have written it with a view to corroborate the correct way (of nurturing the aged).

Treatise on Being Tender Toward the Young

As one approaches 16 years of human life, both the blood and qi are exuberant like the rising sun or the moon grown nearly full. Only yin has not yet grown to be sufficient, and the stomach and intestines are still fragile and narrow. (Therefore, one) must be careful about the *dao* of nurturing (the young).

---

[14] This was a title given to noble women whose husbands were high-ranking officials.

Children should not be clothed in fur and silk. This is a maxim left by past sages which still rings in the ears. The trousers are an article of clothing for the lower part, and silk is much softer than (flax or cotton) cloth. The lower part governs yin, and, when it is exposed to cold and coolness, yin grows easily. But when it is exposed to warmth, yin is whittled away in the dark (*i.e.*, without notice). Therefore, it is really pertinent advice that one should not wear warm silk-padded trousers on the lower part for fear that yin qi should be hindered.

When blood and qi are both exuberant, food is easy to disperse, and, as a result, (children) eat at no (set) times (*i.e.*, frequently. However,) because their stomach and intestines are still fragile and narrow, those (foods) which are thick, sticky, dry, hard, sour, salty, sweet, or pungent, (including) all kinds of fish, meat, fruit, sodden flour (foods), as well as foods that are prepared by roasting, baking, stewing, or frying, (in a word,) any kind of substance that generates heat or is difficult to transform are best prohibited and abstained from. (Children) may be given only dried persimmons, cooked vegetables, and porridge. (Thus,) not only does no disease arise, but the mouth will not be spoilt. (In addition,) virtue is cultivated. Also, raw chestnuts are salty in flavor and dried persimmons are cool in nature. (Therefore,) they can assist in nurturing yin. Nevertheless, because chestnuts, which (granted) supplement greatly, and persimmons, which are astringent, are both difficult to transform, they should only be given in small quantities.

(Some) women are ignorant and know nothing better than to appease (their children's desires). Out of fear the child may cry, they deny it nothing. (However,) when accumulation has developed into an inveterate illness, it is too late to repent. Therefore, it is natural that those rich and noble who dote and coddle (their young) have only children stricken by illness, (and) when (these) grow up, they are soft and tender in sinews and bones. When diseased, they cannot obey the commandments of the mouth to nurture themselves. During the time of mourning, they can not bear a vegetarian diet in order to pay their due respect to the dead (predecessor). Not only are they negligent of small (*i.e.*, personal) matters, but they also fall short of the cardinal principle of righteousness. How can one not be prudent?

As for the breast-feeding mother, it is particularly necessary (for her) to act carefully and with self-restraint. After food and drink is swallowed down, the breast milk flows. If a sexual urge stirs the center, the milk vessels respond. When disease qi reaches the breasts, the milk must congeal and stagnate. If the child receives this kind of milk, disease and illness of either vomiting or diarrhea, sores or heat come in no time. It may be oral putrescence, fright tugging, night crying, or abdominal pain. When the disease first comes on, the urine is invariably very scanty. At this, (one) should inquire without delay and mete out a regulating treatment in accordance with the signs. If the mother is sound, (the child) will also be sound. (Thus the mother's health) may rid (the child) of affliction before it takes shape. The choice of food and drink is comparatively a small matter. In terms of the breast-feeding mother, whether her physique is thick or thin, her temper is moderate or quick, her bones are strong or fragile, her morals are good or bad, the child assimilates (these) rapidly, (and they all) are of particularly great significance.

Some may say, "So that's that!" But I should say, "Not yet

finished!" The ancient (concepts of) fetal education[15] still stand out in the medical books. Therefore, my dull self needs not repeat (these. Nonetheless,) when a fetus in the womb, for example, is caused a disease, the incident arises in the dark. (Thus) people tend to neglect it and physicians are unaware of it. While the child is in the uterus, it shares the same body with its mother. When there is heat, both become hot. When there is cold, both become cold. If there is disease, both are diseased. If healing occurs, both recuperate. (For that reason,) the mother should take particular prudence and care about her food and drink as well as her daily life activities.

The second son of Advanced Scholar[16] Zhang of Dong Yang, aged two, had sores all over (his) head. (These) sores had unexpectedly healed by themselves one day. Subsequently, (he) contracted phlegm dyspnea. Seeing this, I said, "This is fetal toxins. (But) do not by any means administer (toxin-) resolving disinhibitors." All present were confounded. I went on asking, "What kind of substance did its mother like (best of all) during pregnancy?" Zhang replied, "Acrid, pungent, and hot substances used to be her favorites." Accordingly I orally dictated a formula which consisted of Radix Panacis Ginseng (*Ren Shen*), Fructus Forsythiae Suspensae (*Lian Qiao*), Rhizoma Ligustici Wallichii (*Chuan Xiong*), Rhizoma Coptidis Chinensis (*Huang Lian*), raw Radix Glycyrrhizae (*Sheng Gan Cao*), Pericarpium Citri Reticulatae (*Chen Pi*), Radix Paeoniae

---

[15]   The doctrine of fetal education is an ancient one within Chinese medicine. According to this belief, the child *in utero* is influenced by everything their mother experiences. This can include such things as the mother's food as well as her health and disease. It can also include mental and emotional experiences as well. Thus the child's character and temperament are believed to be influenced or educated in the womb by what the mother sees, hears, thinks, and feels as well.

[16]   This title refers to a successful candidate in the imperial examinations.

Lactiflorae (*Shao Yao*), and Caulis Akebiae Mutong (*Mu Tong*). These were to be boiled into a thick decoction and taken with Succus Bambusae (*Zhu Li*) put in boiling water. Several days later, (the patient) was at ease. Some may ask what underlay the diagnosis (*i.e.*, how the condition was diagnosed). My explanation is that since (the child's) essence spirit appeared clouded and fatigued with the disease deeply imbedded yet with no (signs of) external contraction at all, what on earth could it be if not fetal toxins?

My second daughter, who was thin of form and quick-tempered, had had heat in the body in the past. She happened to be in the third month of pregnancy when it was hot summer. She was thirsty and desired water (and) occasionally had a slight fever. I told her to take *Si Wu Tang* (Four Materials Decoction) plus Radix Scutellariae Baicalensis (*Huang Qin*), Pericarpium Citri Reticulatae (*Chen Pi*), raw Radix Glycyrrhizae (*Sheng Gan Cao*), and Caulis Akebiae Mutong (*Mu Tong*). Because she did not feel like boiling (medicinal herbs), she discontinued (the prescription) after (taking only) a couple of doses. Afterwards, when this child of hers was two years old, they suffered from sores all over (their) body. One day the sores healed all of a sudden, and, a few days later, malaria developed. I said, "This is fetal toxins. When the sores recur, the disease will be certainly healed." Later my words turned true. Had (she) kept on the preceding formula in pregnancy, what kind of disease could have occurred (to the child)?

Again, a girl of a Chen family was taken with the disease of epilepsy at eight years (old). When it was rainy or (if she) experienced fright, she would have a fit, foaming at the mouth and crying like a bleating sheep. Having examined (her), I said, "It seems that fright was contracted in the womb." The disease was deeply imbedded and inveterate, but half a year of balancing treatment might cure it. In any case, it was necessary to take bland flavored (food) to assist in establishing the medicinal feat. (I) administered *Shao Dan Yuan* (Burn the Cinnabar Origin)[17] and (later) succeeded it with *Si Wu Tang* with Rhizoma Coptidis Chinensis (*Huang Lian*) added. (During the course of medication,) additions and subtractions were made in accordance with the seasons. Half a year later, (the patient) was at ease.

Treatise on Yin Hidden Internally in the Summer Months

Heaven and earth transform and produce the ten thousand things from one source qi. That (qi) which is rooted in the center is called the divine mechanism, while that which is rooted in the external is called qi and blood. This (same) qi is common among the ten thousand things. Humanity is superior to (other living) things in intelligence. Its form resonates with heaven and earth so that (the three) form a trinity.[18] This is because the qi humanity acquires is righteous and communicates (with heaven and earth). Therefore, (human) qi ascends, floats, descends, and sinks with (the qi of heaven and earth). Humanity shares the one same pair of bellows with heaven and earth.

---

[17]   This consists of Glauberitum (*Xuan Jing Shi*), Calomelas (*Qing Fen*), purified Calomelas (*Fen Shuang*), and Borax (*Peng Sha*).

[18]   Heaven, humanity, and earth form a trinity in traditional Chinese cosmology called the *San Cai* or Three Abilities or Powers.

In the *zi* (B1) month[19], one yang[20] is generated. (This is known as) yang first moving. In the *yin* (B3) month, three yang are generated. This is yang first emerging from the earth. It is the ascension of qi. In the *si* (B6) month, six yang are generated, all yang having emerged to the above. This is the floating of qi. The abdomen of human beings is ascribed to earthly qi. By now, (the earthly qi) is floating in the muscular exterior, dissipating in the skin and hair, and the abdomen is left vacuous.

The classic states:

> In the summer months the channels are filled up (and) earthly qi, spilling and brimming, enters the channels and connecting vessels. Receiving blood (in great amounts), the skin is replenished.

In long summer, qi is in the muscles and flesh, accounting for exterior repletion. When the exterior is replete, the interior is certain to be vacuous. It is popularly known that in the summer months yin is hidden in the internal. This word yin carries the meaning of vacuity. Viewing it as yin cold is a gross error. Some may argue, "When felt with the hand, the abdomen is cold beyond doubt. How can it be otherwise than cold? To treat summerheat disorders, the predecessors

---

[19]   The *zi* month is the eleventh month; the *yin* month is the first month; and the *si* month is the fourth month.

[20]   One yang may also be called the first yang, *i.e.*, *shao yang*, while three yang or the third yang refers to *tai yang*. However, this term can also be understood another way. The former means a small yang qi, while the latter implies exuberant yang qi. The latter interpretation is apparently what is meant in this context since the six yang mentioned in a later place must refer to all yang qi or consummate yang.

had *Yu Long Wan* (Jade Dragon Pills)[21], *Da Shun San* (Great Normalizing Powder)[22], *Gui Ling Wan* (Cinnamomum & Poria Pills)[23], boiled single ingredient Rhizoma Alpiniae Officinari (*Liang Jiang*), *Suo Pi Yin* (Condense the Spleen Drink)[24] comprised of Fructus Amomi Tsao-ko (*Cao Guo*), etc. All of these are formulas to exert warmth and heat. How thoughtless you are!"

To this I should like to reply: In spring and summer, yang should be nurtured. Supreme Servant Wang instructed to eat the cool in spring and the cold in summer so as to nurture yang. His meaning is obvious. (Take) cool platforms, pools of water, big fans, windmills, yin water, cold springs, frozen fruit, and freezing ice. The damage caused by these affects from the internal to the external. If warm and hot (formulas) are not used, how can the disease be overcome? A meticulous musing on the meaning (however,) will reveal that (warm and hot formulas) are not employed really for the sake of hidden yin in the internal.

In addition, the past sages instructed that one should follow

---

21   This consists of Sulphur (*Liu Huang*), Talcum (*Hua Shi*), Mirabilitum (*Xiao Shi*), and Alum (*Ming Fan*).

22   This is composed of Radix Glycyrrhizae (*Gan Cao*), dry Rhizoma Zingiberis (*Gan Jiang*), Semen Pruni Armeniacae (*Xing Ren*), and Cortex Cinnamomi (*Rou Gui*).

23   This consists of Ramulus Cinnamomi (*Gui Zhi*) and Sclerotium Poriae Cocos (*Fu Ling*).

24   This is composed of Fructus Amomi (*Sha Ren*), Fructus Pruni Mume (*Wu Mei*), Fructus Amomi Tsao-ko (*Cao Guo*), mix-fried Radix Glycyrrhizae (*Zhi Gan Cao*), Radix Puerariae Lobatae (*Ge Gen*), and Semen Dolichoris Lablabis (*Bian Dou*).

(qi) in ascension, descension, floating, and sinking but should act counter to cold, heat, warmth, and coolness. Suppose one prescribes without warrant warm and hot (medicinals) in the summer months when fire prevails. How (then) can the mishap of replenishing repletion and evacuating vacuity be avoided?

Some may argue, "As far as the *si* (B6) month is concerned when there is pure yang, (your argument) sounds plausible. The fifth month sees one yin and the sixth month sees two yin. Then how can (summerheat disorders) be other than yin cold?" My reply is: (In these two months) yin is just beginning to move underground, while four yang are floating above the earth, burning and blazing, scorching and incinerating, with metal liquified and rock melted. Where is yin cold? Immortal Sun[25] designed *Sheng Mai San* (Generate the Pulse Powder) and bid people to take (this) in the summer months. What is it for if not for vacuity?

Treatise on Master Chen's Formulary for Pox Sores

When reading books by predecessors, it is necessary to grasp the meaning of their writings. If while reading a book one does not try to grasp its meaning but just searches for (some) appropriate application, one will gain nothing (in their

---

[25] The Immortal Sun refers to Sun Si-miao, the most famous Chinese doctor of the Tang dynasty and author of the *Qian Jin Yao Fang* (*Prescriptions [Worth] A Thousand [Pieces of] Gold*).

search). As regards pox sores, Master Qian[26] has given a most detailed discussion. Comprehensively discoursing on the origin and development (of this condition and) the (involved) channels and connecting vessels, clearly identifying the exterior and the interior, vacuity and repletion, illustrating at length the treatment methods, quoting as substantiation the statements and arguments (from the classics), he elaborated a monumental style of writing and bequeathing instructions to posterity. After reading (his work), a learner is able to apply it to practice as if drawing a circle and square with compass and ruler or determining an even (surface) or straight (line) with a yardstick. Enabled to make inference and extension, analogy and stretching, (the reader) can augment (the knowledge contained in this book) and put it to inexhaustible use.

Nowadays, (some) people who are ignorant of the cause of disease and do not seek the implication in the design of a formula, try a formula casually after picking it out in a hurry (merely) based on its indicated pattern. If it fails to induce a (positive) response, they give it up together with the book (containing it). This (behavior) is too thoughtless. Recently, because the teachings of the *Ju Fang* have been in vogue for long and the theory of the *Su Wen* has been forsaken, those persons who prate about medicine (merely) in terms of their

---

[26]   The Master Qian referred to is Qian Yi, a.k.a. Qian Zhong-yang, circa 1032-1113 CE. Born in Yun Zhou, now Dong Ping in Shandong Province, Qian Yi was a distinguished pediatrician who was appointed court physician in 1090 CE. Having specialized in pediatrics for more than 40 years, his student, Yan Xiao-zhong, collected and edited his writings in the book *Xiao Er Yao Zheng Zhi Jue (The Key to Medicinals in Pediatric Disease)*. This was one of the earliest books in Chinese specifically on the treatment of infants and children. Qian Yi was the first to emphasize treatment based on pattern differentiation in measles, scarlet fever, smallpox, and chickenpox.

own illness like warm but are averse to cold (formulas. In addition, they) like supplementation but are averse to resolving and disinhibiting. Suddenly, they have come across a treatise on formulas by Master Chen which includes nothing but dry, hot, supplementing formulas. His expression is authoritative and his language is terse. Delighted, they apply it. Of the same mind, they entertain full belief in it, thinking Master Qian to be far inferior to Master Chen.

Some may ask, "Do you assume Master Chen's formulas as defective?" My answer is, "Though he does deserve mention for being good at tracing disease conditions, Master Chen's formulas are truly biased towards one single principle. Largely, his idea is to ascribe (pox sores) to and focus (their treatment) on one single channel, the *tai yin*. The hand *tai yin* is ascribed to the lungs (which) govern the skin and hair. The foot *tai yin* is ascribed to the spleen (and) governs the muscles and flesh. Lung metal is averse to cold and liable to contract (it), while spleen stomach earth is averse to dampness and denies no reception to anything. According to his use of Flos Caryophylli (*Ding Xiang*) and Cortex Cinnamomi (*Guan Gui*), he (aims at) treating cold in the lungs, (while) his use of Radix Praeparatus Aconiti Carmichaeli (*Fu Zi*), Rhizoma Atractylodis Macrocephalae (*Bai Zhu*), and Rhizoma Pinelliae Ternatae (*Ban Xia*, aims at) treating dampness in the spleen. If cold does indeed exist in the lungs and dampness in the spleen with vacuity in addition, administration (of these medicinals) with discretion will certainly hit and terminate the disease. There will definitely be no hurt brought on.

Now picture another situation. Whenever (people) see a case of retarded eruption of sores, body heat, diarrhea, fright palpitation, qi urgency, or thirst and desire for drink, they indiscriminately prescribe *Mu Xiang San* (Saussurea Powder)

31

and *Yi Gong San* (Wonder Working Powder)[27] regardless of whether (the disease) is cold or heat, vacuity or repletion. Occasionally, they hit upon (the disease) and presently achieve an effect. (But) suppose (such formulas) are abused. Disaster will follow upon the heels (of their administration).

Why is this? In the prescriptions and formulas designed by the ancients, there were guiding ingredients, preparatory supervision, counterassistance, and use of the cause.[28] In Master Qian's formulary, it is true that Herba Cum Radice Asari Sieboldi (*Xi Xin*), Flos Caryophylli (*Ding Xiang*), Rhizoma Atractylodis Macrocephalae (*Bai Zhu*), Radix Panacis Ginseng (*Ren Shen*), Radix Astragali Membranacei (*Huang Qi*), etc. are not abandoned (altogether). However, usually there are supervisors and assistants (in Master Qian's formulas) which do not exclusively implement warm supplementation. Master Qian (tended to) use many cool and cold (medicinals). But as for the adjuvant and assistant method, he just gave a preliminary touch without going deep (in his writings). There is no point in telling dreams before an idiot. Although Master Qian was extremely solicitous, he (nevertheless) expected those who were enlightened to expand and augment (his formulary) in practice.

Although Master Chen distinctly surpassed his predecessors as the inventor of employing warm medicinals in the case of

---

[27]   This is composed of Radix Panacis Ginseng (*Ren Shen*), Sclerotium Poriae Cocos (*Fu Ling*), Rhizoma Atractylodis Macrocephalae (*Bai Zhu*), Pericarpium Citri Reticulatae (*Chen Pi*), and Radix Glycyrrhizae (*Gan Cao*).

[28]   Use of the cause or *yin yong* is a technical term in Chinese herbal medicine. It refers to processing a medicinal with a method that is the same nature as the cause of disease. For instance, a cold medicinal used to clear heat may be processed by heat, such as by stir-frying.

thirst and supplementing ones in the case of itchy and sunken (poxes), much use of dry, hot medicinals, such as Cortex Cinnamomi (*Gui*), Radix Praeparatus Aconiti Carmichaeli (*Fu*), and Flos Caryophylli (*Ding Xiang*), is probably inappropriate. Why? Cortex Cinnamomi, Radix Praeparatus Aconiti Carmichaeli, Flos Caryophylli, and the like are truly necessary and appropriate if cold and vacuity exist. (But) if there is vacuity perhaps with no cold, what harm they will bring! When designing a formula based on Master Chen, it is truly proper to employ supplementation with dry, hot (medicinals), but only if there is cold contained in the pox sores. Now if there is no cold contained, but (people) use biased formulas (of this kind), then are (such formulas) not excessively hot? I have been gathering the pith and essence from various masters and trying to implement their meaning in practice. (Yet) I have never dared to base myself on a ready formula of theirs. Let me cite one or two examples as proof.

My nephew suffered from pox sores at the age of six or seven with fever, slight thirst, and loose stools. A pediatrician received him and prescribed *Mu Xiang San* with 10 pieces of Flos Caryophylli (*Ding Xiang*) added per dose. I was extremely skeptical (of this approach. The progression of the pox) were observed to be retarded. This was indeed because of loose bowels and qi weakness. The stools were found to be all stinking, stagnated, old, and accumulated (substances). This kind of stools are due to hot steaming of the stomach and intestines rather than to existence of cold and vacuity. (I) promptly stopped (the formula), but one dose had already been administered. Subsequently, (I) prescribed *Huang Lian Jie Du Tang* (Coptis Resolve Toxins Decoction) with Rhizoma Atractylodis Macrocephalae (*Bai Zhu*) added. In order to resolve the heat of Flos Caryophylli, 10 doses were administered. Then diarrhea was checked and (the pox) sores erupted. Later, there was constantly slight heat in his muscles, and *yong* boils grew on his hands and feet. Over one month of balancing and supplementation with cool medicinals (and the patient was) at ease.

Again, a male aged 16-17 had fever with cloudedness and loss of vision and hearing. The pulses on both hands were hollow, large, and a little rapid. (I) realized that he was damaged by taxation. At the time, many in (his) neighborhood were taken with pox. Although he was unable to recognize people, he drank medicine and ate gruel when given. Then I instructed (his family) to administer a large dose of a thick decoction boiled from Radix Panacis Ginseng (*Ren Shen*), Radix Astragali Membranacei (*Huang Qi*), Radix Angelicae Sinensis (*Dang Gui*), Rhizoma Atractylodis Macrocephalae (*Bai Zhu*), and Pericarpium Citri Reticulatae (*Chen Pi*). Not till over 30 doses were drunk did the pox erupt. Another 20 odd doses and they became purulent with no skin intact anywhere over the body.

Some asked, "Since the disease developed in a threatening way, why should not a complete formula from Master Chen be used for the treatment?" I answered: This was nothing but vacuity and without cold, and, (therefore,) the preceding formula should be insisted on. Then tens of doses more issued in recovery. Afterwards, (when) the patient was asked about the cause of his disease, he said that four or five days before (the disease), for fear that a pox disease should arise, he strained himself hard by cutting firewood and sweated copiously for days in succession. If a complete formula of Master Chen had been used, what a cause for repentance would this have been?

In the spring of the *jia shen* year (*i.e.,* 1344), during the reign of Zhi Zheng[29], yang qi started earlier than usual. In the first month, pox sores spread, never skipping over one household in the country. Because of indiscriminate administration of Master Chen's formulas, more than a hundred children and infants lost their lives. Although (this disaster) was predetermined by heavenly number[30], I am afraid that human behavior which was not satisfactory must also be held responsible.

Treatise on Painful Wind

Qi travels outside the vessels, while blood travels inside the vessels. By day, they travel 25 circuits in the yang. By night, they travel another 25 circuits in yin. This is because normal people are so created and transformed. Subject to cold, they travel slowly and become insufficient. Subject to heat, they travel fast and become excessive. If the internal is damaged by the seven affects and the external is damaged by the six qi, blood and qi may circulate either fast or slow, giving rise to disease.

In those with painful wind, (this condition) is usually caused at first by blood heated to a boil. Later, because of wading in

---

[29] This was the reign name of Emperor Shun Di of the Yuan dynasty, 1341-1368 CE.

[30] Heavenly number refers to the Chinese system of astrology utilizing the celestial stems and terrestrial branches to identify cycles of change within the phenomenal world. This system was, in fact, more of a numerology.

cold water, standing on damp ground, fanning for coolness, or sleeping in a draught, cold and coolness gather externally. When hot blood meets with this cold, it becomes turbid, congealed, and stagnated, thus causing pain. This pain gets worse at night because (qi and blood) are traveling in the yin. The treatment method consists of using acrid, hot medicinals to flow and dissipate cold dampness, and open and effuse the interstices. When blood is able to circulate and becomes harmonious with qi, the disease will certainly heal. There are, however, more than one treatment method (and these) are somewhat different. (I) will write (about) one or two of them by way of illustration.

Fu Wen of Dong Yang was over 60 years of age. He was quick of temper and taxed by toiling. He suffered from severe pain in the legs which became worse with movement. Having examined (him), I said that this was a pattern complicated by vacuity. It was necessary to supplement and warm the blood, and then the disease would naturally heal. Accordingly, (I) prescribed *Si Wu Tang* (Four Materials Decoction) plus Semen Pruni Persicae (*Tao Ren*), Pericarpium Citri Reticulatae (*Chen Pi*), Radix Achyranthis Bidentatae (*Niu Xi*), and raw Radix Glycyrrhizae (*Sheng Gan Cao*. These) were boiled. Then raw Rhizoma Zingiberis (*Sheng Jiang*) and ground *Qian Xing San* (Lurking Powder)[31] were put in (and the decoction) was taken hot. Thirty to 40 doses and (the patient) was at ease.

Again, the wife of a Zhu family, aged nearly 30, used to eat very thick flavored (foods) and had an impetuous and quick temper. She suffered from painful wind with contracture for

---

[31] This is composed of Cortex Phellodendri (*Huang Bai*) which is soaked in wine, dried, and powdered. It is taken with Succus Zingiberis (*Jiang Zhi*).

several months. (Attending) physicians prayed with no response (*i.e.*, tried in vain). Having examined (her), I said that this was a pattern with phlegm and qi contained. It was necessary to harmonize the blood, course the qi, and conduct phlegm. Then the disease would naturally heal. Accordingly, (I) prescribed *Qian Xing San* with the introduction of raw Radix Glycyrrhizae (*Sheng Gan Cao*), Radix Achyranthis Bidentatae (*Niu Xi*), mix-fried Fructus Citri Seu Ponciri (*Zhi Qiao*), Medulla Tetrapanacis Papyriferi (*Tong Cao*), Pericarpium Citri Reticulatae (*Chen Pi*), Semen Pruni Persicae (*Tao Ren*), and Succus Zingiberis (*Jiang Zhi*. These) were boiled and taken. Half a year later, (the patient) was at ease.

Again, a neighbor, Bao Liu, aged over 20, had been given astringing medicinals in order to affect his bloody dysentery. Later he contracted painful wind, crying and shouting so loudly that the houses in (his) neighborhood shook. Having examined (him), I said that this was a pattern of malign blood entering the channels and connecting vessels. Blood, if subjected to damp heat, over time will certainly become congealed and turbid. As it had not been completely precipitated, it was retained and stagnated in the tunnels, thus giving pain. If it were not treated (properly) for long, it well might develop into hemilateral withering. Accordingly, (I) prescribed tens of doses of *Si Wu Tang* plus Semen Pruni Persicae (*Tao Ren*), Flos Carthami Tinctorii (*Hong Hua*), Radix Achyranthis Bidentatae (*Niu Xi*), Radix Scutellariae Baicalensis (*Huang Qin*), Pericarpium Citri Reticulatae (*Chen Pi*), and raw Radix Glycyrrhizae (*Sheng Gan Cao*. These) were boiled and raw Rhizoma Zingiberis (*Sheng Jiang*) and ground *Qian Xing San* were put in. This was drunk with a small amount of wine. In addition, (I) pricked Bend Middle (*Wei Zhong*, Bl 40).

Nearly three *he*[32] of blackish blood was let out, and (the patient) was at ease.

Some may ask, "(We) have often seen neighbors drink wine with ground medicinal herbs put in, and sometimes no more than a (small) number of doses have achieved a cure. As you have explained, it took all the (above) cases a long time to show effect. Is this not too circuitous and slow?" My answer is that those disease-thwarting herbal medicinals, (for example,) *Shi Shang Cai Shi Si*[33] used as the sovereign and Rhizoma Smilacis Glabrae (*Guo Shan Long*) and the like as assistants, are all hot and dry in nature. (They are) able to dry dampness but not nurture yin. In the case of a shallow disease, where damp phlegm can be opened when met with dryness and hot blood is able to circulate when met with heat, they may possibly achieve some effect. For those with deep disease and scant blood, the more thwarting (medicinals) are used, the more vacuity there will be. (Further,) the more thwarting (medicinals), the more deeply (the disease penetrates. The above-discussed) Zhu was such a case. Then do you still think I am circuitous and slow?

---

[32]   1 *he* equals 1/10 liter.

[33]   We have not been able to identify this medicinal. Its name literally means stone fiber picked on the rock. It may be Herba Elatostemae Umbellati.

Treatise on Quartan Ague

The *Nei Jing* states, "If (one) is damaged by heat in summer and by wind in autumn, (one) will unavoidably be taken with malarial disease." Quartan ague is (so-called) old malaria. Because it attacks every third day and hangs on persistently, it acquires such a name. The past sages have left (some) treatment methods (for this) which are all harsh formulas. (However,) some of these are not appropriate for those with a constitution of a weak nature or those affected by (an inappropriate way of) living and nurturing. Only Master Xu included in his formulas supplementing medicinals like Radix Panacis Ginseng (*Ren Shen*) and Radix Astragali Membranacei (*Huang Qi*). However, because he did not attach a detailed discussion, it is difficult for later students to conjecture (the proper use of these medicinals).

In recent years, the majority of people become feeble and weak before 50 years of age. Moreover, those overindulgent in dietary and sexual desires without any self-restraint are ten times more (in number). If (one has) a weak physique but is taken by a deep disease, it is most difficult to prescribe medication. (In view of this situation,) I began to realize that if Radix Dichroae (*Chang Shan*), Fructus Pruni Mume (*Wu Mei*), Arsenic (*Pi Dan*), etc., all of which are medicinals to thwart phlegm, are misused, a minor disorder will become serious, and a serious disease is bound to end in death.

Why is this? Attacking every three days indicates that yin is subject to disease. (Malaria) attacking on the days of *zi* (B1), *wu* (B7), *mao* (B4), and *you* (B10) is *shao yin* malaria. (That) attacking on the days of *yin* (B3), *shen* (B9), *si* (B6), and *hai*

(B12) is *jue yin* malaria. (And that) attacking on the days of *chen* (B5), *xu* (B11), *chou* (B2), and *wei* (B8) is *tai yin* malaria.

Malaria contracted as a result of summerheat should be resolved with diaphoresis. (In enjoying coolness) on a cool platform, in the water pavilion, in the shade of trees, on the cold ground, when being fanned by someone else, or having a bath in a spring, the sweat cannot be discharged and is depressed into phlegm. At the initial stage of contraction, the stomach qi is still strong enough (for one) not to be conscious of it at all. Even if a second contraction occurs, one is still ignorantly unaware and may continue to take drink and food to their heart's content. They may overtax, toil, and strain themselves in chamber affairs (*i.e.*, sexual intercourse. Consequently,) stomach qi is greatly damaged and there arises disease. This disease is deep-rooted and firmly fixed. Because it is, for this reason, very difficult to cure, patients are (all the more) eager for rapid recovery, and physicians, eager for an immediate gain, recklessly prescribe sweet, acrid, harsh formulas. What they are ignorant of is that affection by wind and affection by summerheat are both exterior evils which should be resolved through diaphoresis. Since the affection is deep, it absolutely cannot be eliminated by one or two *sheng* of (exuded) sweat.

There are also cases where the stomach qi has recovered a little and spontaneous sweating already appears, but, because of failure to abide by the prohibitions and commandments, (patients) are subjected to and offended by new (evils). While old evils are not yet removed, new ones are contracted. Progressing sinuously, settling and stagnating, the disease penetrates more deeply. In addition, those coming for treatment are all only too willing to try (a remedy of supposedly) quick effect. However, these disease-thwarting medicinals can bring severe damage to their stomach qi. I know that (such patients) can hardly avoid a disastrous end.

Therefore, I would rather be slow and dull and decelerate my pace. It is necessary first to prescribe supplementing medicinals, such as Radix Panacis Ginseng (*Ren Shen*), Rhizoma Atractylodis Macrocephalae (*Bai Zhu*), Pericarpium Citri Reticulatae (*Chen Pi*), and Radix Paeoniae Lactiflorae (*Shao Yao*), and to assist these with medicinals pertinent to the involved channel with only a view to inducing perspiration. If perspiration is induced but the body turns vacuous, then it is necessary to employ large amounts of supplementing medicinals as assistants. Only when perspiration exits all over the body, passing beyond Bend Middle (*Wei Zhong*, Bl 40), is it a propitious sign. Even then, (I) still instruct (the patient) to try to be indifferent to food and drink, to seldom go out, to take shelter from wind and prefer a warm (place), and to stay away from the bed curtains. (If one) takes meticulous care about regulating and nurturing, recuperation will never fail to follow.

Suppose the disease is contracted deeply. Although a massive sweat is induced and the contracted evil must be transmitted out from the viscera to the bowels, its attack will inevitably become erratic and irregular. Is this still a propitious sign? To treat this kind of disease is easy in spring and summer, but difficult in autumn and winter. Except for (the degree of) easiness or difficulty in (promoting) diaphoresis, nothing (else) is (the criterion for) the superiority or inferiority (of a treatment).

It may be asked, "There are not a few ancient formulas which include Arsenic (*Pi Dan*), Fructus Pruni Mume (*Wu Mei*), and Radix Dichroae (*Chang Shan*), and they have proven effective. Do you not think them to be usable?" My answer is that when the bowels are subjected to disease, (malaria) is shallow, attacking once a day. Attacks every other day (show that) the stomach qi is still strong. (Therefore, those formulas) can be administered anyway. If it attacks every three days, the disease is already in the viscera. Disease existing in the viscera is difficult to treat. As an external contraction, it may be curable. Yet (one) can never expect a rapid effect through employing thwarting medicinals.

Honorable[34] Zhan, Secretary of the Provincial Prosecutor, aged nearly 60, had very robust physique, very strong form, and very somber complexion. Last year, (he) contracted quartan ague in the second month. I was sent over for an examination. Aware that he used to have plenty of rich, fat (food), I told him that he should keep away from beauty's charm and have a bland diet. A whole month of regulating and rectifying would bring about a massive perspiration and recovery would follow. (At this,) the lord was displeased. A person beside (him) said that (the disease) was easy (to treat) and could be cured in a couple of days. (He thus) prescribed a thwarting formula. Three to five doses (taken) and the disease abated. (However,) 10 days after, it arose again. (The same formula) was administered once more, and (the malaria) abated once more. Thus the disease lingered till winter when it remained yet to be removed. (The lord) came to me for a treatment again. I knew he had been taking medication for long and had little phlegm, but his stomach qi was not completely exhausted. Moreover, owing to the cold weather, perspiration was not thoroughly induced. Therefore, I prescribed pills mixed with gruel made of two *jin* of Rhizoma Atractylodis Macrocephalae (*Bai Zhu*) and bid

---

[34] The title *sui* means revered or honorable. This word also means both public and impartial. As a term of respect for a public official, it obviously implies more than reverence.

him, when hungry, not to take any food for the time being but 100-200 of these pills with hot boiled water. (He should also) have nothing but rice gruel to regulate and nurture (the stomach). When the medicine was consumed, a copious sweating would be induced and recovery follow. Later on my words turned true. There have been many (successful) cases like this. Only the medicinal varied in amounts. There is no need to describe all these cases.

Treatise on Not Attacking Those with Damaged Stomach Qi in Spite of Replete Disease Evil

When discussing how to rule the country, (people) usually borrow (the practice of) medicine as a metaphor. How humanitarian their statements are! The true qi is the people, whereas disease evils are bandits and robbers. Whenever there are bandits and robbers, they must be wiped out before (public) safety can be ensured. Before taking action, competent ministers and generals must first calculate the vacuity and repletion of military forces and rations and the pros and cons of the situation. If actions are taken rashly and recklessly, the people will first have a hard time with the bandits and then (secondly) with the (armed) forces. When the people have a hard time, the country becomes weak. Taking adventurous action and leaving things to chance is the behavior of a base person. There are tens of thousands of things interwoven in the universe, and they definitely carry evident retributions between them. How can one not take this to heart? (Thus) please allow (me) to cite one or two examples.

Lu of Yong Kang[35], a relative (of mine) who was thin in form and (had) a black complexion, was addicted to wine his entire life. (Yet he) was never intoxicated even after having drunk quantities (of alcohol). He was nearly half a 100 years old, supporting concubines (besides his wife). One day, he suddenly had a fit of quivering with great aversion to cold, declaring of thirst yet drinking no water. I felt his pulse which was large and weak but, in the right *guan* section, somewhat replete and a little rapid and choppy when pressure was applied. Accordingly, (I) determined (his condition was one of) wine heat depressed internally and unable to drain out due to exterior heat with no vacuity. (For this,) one single medicinal, Radix Astragali Membranacei (*Huang Qi*), was boiled in a soup of dry Radix Puerariae Lobatae (*Gan Ge*) and taken. When two *liang* of Astragalus and one *liang* of Pueraria were consumed, great perspiration was obtained. The next morning (he) was at ease.

Elder Born[36] She suffered from stagnant sensation diarrhea with severe pressure in (his) rectum, the very pattern for which *Cheng Qi Tang* (Support the Qi Decoction)[37] is indicat-

---

[35]   This is the name of a place near to the home town of the author.

[36]   *Xian sheng* literally translates as elder born in Chinese. However, it means gentleman, sir, teacher, or an educated person. In modern Chinese it is the equivalent of Mister.

[37]   This is a collective term for *Da, Xiao,* and *Tiao Wei Cheng Qi Tang* (Major, Minor & Balance the Stomach Support the Qi Decoctions). The major is composed of Radix Et Rhizoma Rhei (*Da Huang*), Cortex Magnoliae Officinalis (*Hou Po*), Fructus Immaturus Citri Seu Ponciri (*Zhi Shi*), Mirabilitum (*Mang Xiao*), and mix-fried Radix Glycyrrhizae (*Zhi Gan Cao*). The minor consists of stir-fried Cortex Magnoliae Officinalis (*Hou Po*) and stir-fried Fructus Immaturus Citri Seu Ponciri (*Zhi Shi*). The stomach-balancing one consists of Radix Et Rhizoma

44

ed. I said, since the qi opening pulse was vacuous with form replete but (his) facial complexion was yellow and somewhat white, this (condition) was definitely due to overeating in the past damaging the stomach. (He) would have to bear the trouble and affliction for a day or two (before a cure was affected. I) prescribed more than 10 doses of Radix Panacis Ginseng (*Ren Shen*), Rhizoma Atractylodis Macrocephalae (*Bai Zhu*), Pericarpium Citri Reticulatae (*Chen Pi*), Radix Paeoniae Lactiflorae (*Shao Yao*), and some other supplementing medicinals. Three days later, (his) stomach qi was a little mended. (Then) two doses of *Cheng Qi (Tang)* was administered and (he was) at ease. If *Cheng Qi (Tang)* had been rashly administered before the damage of the stomach qi had been mended by supplementation, even though the disease had recovered, I am afraid (he) could not have avoided becoming thin and exhausted.

A maiden servant, aged nearly 40, (had) a purplish complexion and was a little fat. (She) was reflective in character (and) liable to worry. Her menses had been absent for three months, and there was a qi mass in the middle of her lower abdomen. Initially, it had been the size of a chestnut, but gradually it had grown to the size of a cake. I palpated her pulse which was choppy and heavy (*i.e.*, sluggish) on both hands but present[38] when pressure was applied. The mass was acutely painful when (I) tried to press (it), and it seemed on palpation to be one half *cun* above (the surrounding skin. I) prescribed *Xiao Shi Wan* (Niter Pills) from the *Qian Jin ([Formulas {Worth}] a Thousand [Pieces of] Gold)*. After four to five times (of this treatment), she unexpectedly informed

---

Rhei (*Da Huang*), mix-fried Radix Glycyrrhizae (*Zhi Gan Cao*), and Mirabilitum (*Mang Xiao*).

[38] The translator suspects absent should be read for present.

(me) that her nipples had turned black and contained breast milk and that she might be pregnant. I said that was not so. A choppy pulse is a definite argument against pregnancy. (I, therefore,) prescribed three to five more doses, and the pulse felt a little vacuous and hollow. I realized that the medicinals were too drastic and bid her to stop the formula.

Then *Si Wu Tang* (Four Materials Decoction) was administered with Rhizoma Atractylodis Macrocephalae (*Bai Zhu*) in double amount and with Pericarpium Citri Reticulatae (*Chen Pi*) added as an assistant. After 30 doses (were taken) and (her) pulse was mended, *Xiao Shi Wan* were administered again. After four to five times (of such treatment), she told (me) abruptly that the mass had dispersed (*i.e.*, shrunk) by a circle. At this (I) told her not to take any more (of the formula). Half a month later, her menses came with severe pain and nearly one half *sheng* of blackish blood precipitated in which there were scores of pepper seed-like clots. By now the mass was dispersed by half and she came for more medication in the hope of eliminating the remaining (part of the) mass. I explained to her that she should not be impatient and that, since the mass was already broken, no more attacking (formula) was allowed. (I further assured her that) the mass would certainly disperse altogether with (her) menstrual flow the next month. The next month when her menses came, small amounts of blackish blood clots were precipitated, and (the mass was) dispersed by another circle. She came once more asking for medication. I assured (her) that if only she abided by the prohibitions and commandments, (the mass) was bound to disperse completely the following month. Later (my words) proved true.

Generally speaking, attacking medicinals are received by disease if there is any. (But) if the disease evil is light and the strength of the medicinals is heavy, they may damage the stomach qi. The stomach qi is a clear, pure, peaceful, and harmonious qi which agrees only with grains, meats, vegetables, and fruits. All medicinal herbs and stones have a qi of biased, overwhelming proclivity. Even Radix Panacis Ginseng (*Ren Shen*) and Radix Astragali Membranacei (*Huang Qi*), are kinds (of medicinals) biased in nature, let alone attacking medicinals. In the above woman, (her) stomach qi was originally weak and, additionally, there was scant good blood. If (attacking) medication had (only) stopped with complete dispersion of the mass, there would have been almost no stomach qi left. If things had been let go so far, could the physician have been called a physician?

Treatise on Observing the Form & Colors Before Examining the Pulse & Inquiring into Signs in the Treatment of Disease

The *Nei Jing* states:

> The *dao* of pulse examination (requires) observing the patient's courage and trepidation and muscles, flesh, and skin before one is able to know the conditions. This is regarded as the (right) method of diagnosis.

Generally speaking, in connection with a person's form, being tall is inferior to being short, being large (is inferior) to being small, and being fat (is inferior) to being thin. In regard to the complexion, white is inferior to black, tenderness to somberness, and thinness to thickness. Furthermore, a fat person is abundant in dampness, while a thin person is abundant in fire. A white (complexion) indicates lung qi vacuity, while a black (one) indicates ample kidney qi. Form and complexion are different (from one person to another), and (therefore) so are the viscera and bowels. (When form and complexion differ, although) the external signs may be (otherwise) much the same, treatment (may) differ diametrically. It follows that, for a fat person, a floating pulse is a treasure, while for a thin person, a deep pulse is a treasure. In the case of an impetuous person, a moderate pulse should arouse suspicion, while in the case of a moderate person, an urgent pulse should arouse suspicion. (This is) because (people) cannot be viewed from the same one angle. Let (me) cite one or two cases which can serve as analogous examples.

Chen (was a) a friend (of mine) in Dong Yang. (He) had prominent sinews and (his) body was a little lanky. He suffered from body vacuity and taxation with headache, and he even had left a deathbed will. I found his pulse to be wiry, large, and rapid. (I) prescribed Radix Panacis Ginseng (*Ren Shen*), Rhizoma Atractylodis Macrocephalae (*Bai Zhu*) as sovereigns and Rhizoma Ligustici Wallichii (*Chuan Xiong*) and Pericarpium Citri Reticulatae (*Chen Pi*) as assistants. Five to six days passed but (his condition) did not improve. Everyone was confused, thinking that the prescription must be incorrect. I said that the medicinals exerted their strength step by step and that (we) should wait for one or two short nights and recovery would naturally result. Unexpectedly, his youngest son came up, asking how about adding a little Radix Astragali Membranacei (*Huang Qi*). I smiled without replying. Another night passed, and (the patient) unexpectedly said that the disease had suddenly been cured. I felt his pulse and found it a little more exuberant under my fingers. After another half day, the patient complained of fullness above the diaphragm and no feeling of hunger. Seeing his

48

abdomen reticulation obscured (*i. e.* seeing his abdomen a little swollen), I asked whether Radix Astragali Membranacei had been added to the decoction since the night before. The answer was yes, but it was added to only three doses. Then (I) prescribed *Er Chen Tang* (Two Aged Decoction) plus Cortex Magnoliae Officinalis (*Hou Po*), Fructus Citri Seu Ponciri (*Zhi Qiao*), Rhizoma Coptidis Chinensis (*Huang Lian*) to drain his defensive (qi). Three doses and he was at ease.

Again, Zheng, a friend of mine in Yi Men, Pu Jiang, aged over 20, ran a high fever in the autumn with thirst and confused speech and vision. The disease looked like (obsession) by an evil ghost. Seven to eight days later, I was sent for treatment. I felt his pulse which was surging, rapid, and replete on both hands and found that his form was fat with a whitish red facial complexion. Luckily his sinews (*i.e.*, veins) were prominent and the root of the pulse was not replete as a result of cool medicinals. This was a disease due to taxation fatigue and would naturally be overcome after administration of warm supplementing medicinals. Seven to eight doses of *Chai Hu (Tang*, Bupleurum Decoction) was said (to have been administered. I) prescribed *Huang Qi Fu Zi Tang* (Astragalus & Aconite Decoction) which was to be taken cooled. After three doses, (he) was sleepy and fatigued, falling into a sound sleep. Resolution followed moderate perspiration with the pulse also becoming a little softened. This was followed by *Huang Qi Bai Zhu Tang* (Astragalus & Atractylodes Decoction). Ten days later, the pulse had gradually contracted and was becoming small. (Therefore,) the administration (of the above) continued. Another half month and (he) was at ease.

Rhizoma Astragali Membranacei (*Huang Qi*) is a qi-supplementing medicinal. Of the above two people, one (case) was (due to) qi vacuity, while the other was (due to) qi repletion.

49

There exist appropriateness and inappropriateness (in using medicinals). How can this not be taken into account?

Treatise on Not Abiding by Prohibitions & Commandments in Great (*i.e.*, Serious) Disease

When diseased, one must take medicine and must abide by (the relevant) prohibitions and commandments. In his *Qian Jin Fang (Prescriptions [Worth] a Thousand [Pieces of] Gold)*, Immortal Sun gave detailed instructions about (such) prohibitions and commandments, but he failed to give a detailed discussion about the reasons for the abiding by (these. Below) I venture to give an outlined discussion (of these) in the form of admonitions.

Human beings depend on the stomach qi for life, it being a clear, pure, peaceful, and harmonious qi. Preoccupation and worry taxing the spirit, labor and activity tormenting the form, sexual desire without restraint, thought and aspiration being frustrated, inappropriate diet, and misused medication, all these may damage (the stomach qi. Once) damaged, it ought to be nurtured and supplemented. If, unperturbed by not knowing what to blame, one continues to wilfully violate the (relevant) prohibitions, the old pattern already inflicted will accumulate (more and more) with each passing day. (In this case,) we might see physicians too busy to receive (their clients, while) there were no hope that the damaged, vanquished stomach qi could recover completely (on its own. Thus) death would be close by.

50

My clan uncle was replete both in form and complexion. (He) suffered from malarial disease as well as dysentery. Relying too much on his sturdy (physique) and (his) ability to eat, undaunted, he defied any prohibition. One day, he sent for me, saying, "Although I am diseased, I am strong and able to eat. However, I feel bitter about (*i.e.*, I am distressed) by the exiting of sweat. Can you stop (this) perspiration?" I answered, "Malarial disease cannot be overcome except through the exiting of sweat. What worries (me) is none other than your being strong and able to eat." This was not dysentery. His stomach, which was hot, was good at dispersing (grains), but his spleen, which was diseased, was unable to transform (these. Therefore,) food accumulation and the disease condition were already very serious. At this juncture, it was necessary to adopt an abstemious and selective diet to nurture the stomach qi and to avoid going out so as to protect from wind and cold. When a thorough sweating was induced, recuperation would follow.

(At this, my) uncle said, "Vulgar (*i. e.* common people) say that there is no death from dysentery with a full stomach. Since I am able to eat, what can be said to worry (about)?" I said, "Dysentery with ability to eat reveals that the stomach qi is not yet diseased. Because of that, no death is spoken of. This statement, however, does not refer to those that eat unscrupulously without abstention and selection." Not following my advice, he continued to devour (his food) unscrupulously, eating plenty of fruit whenever feeling thirsty. More than a month passed in this way. When he (really) intended to be treated, (I) had no means to take (his case) in hand. After lingering for over a month more, he died. The *Nei Jing* considers arrogance, self-indulgence, and unreasonableness to be an incurable disease. This is quite believable!

Another man named Zhou was replete both in form and complexion. (He) had suffered for five days from dysentery with large food intake and rapid hungering. He devoured (his food) without any selectivity. I censured him, saying that during illness one should nurture oneself by balancing and supplementation. How could one allow good flavor to mutilate and plunder oneself? Then (I) told him to eat only gruel with cooked turnip. (I) treated him in a small way by regulating (the stomach) for half a month and he was at ease.

Treatise on Vacuity Disease & Phlegm Disease Resembling Ghost Possession

Blood and qi are the spirit of the body. When the spirit is decrepit and exhausted, (ghost) evils can consequently enter (the body). In truth, this may occur. (However,) if both blood and qi are depleted and phlegm intrudes into the middle burner, obstructing the upbearing and downbearing (of blood and qi, blood and qi) will be unable to transport and function. Thus each of the twelve officials fail to carry on their duties, and vision, hearing, speech, and movement all become vacuous and frenetic. If (this condition) is treated as a (ghost) evil, the patient will surely die. What a wrong which should not have happened will be done! Who should be held responsible for this blunder?

A friend (of mine), Fu, son of the Secretary of the Prosecutor's Yeomen, was 17 or 18 years of age. In a summer month, (he) was thirsty from great taxation and drank quantities of plum juice to his heart's content. In addition, he experienced terrible fright three or four times in succession. As a result, he contracted a disease of confused speech and vision which looked like obsession by an evil ghost. (I) felt his pulse which was vacuous and wiry as well as deep and rapid on both hands. I concluded that a rapid pulse indicated the existence of heat; a vacuous and wiry pulse revealed great fright; and that the plums' sour juice was depressed in the middle venter. Only if vacuity was supplemented, heat cleared, and stagnated phlegm led out would this disease be overcome. Then (I) administered Radix Panacis Ginseng (*Ren Shen*), Rhizoma Atractylodis Macrocephalae (*Bai Zhu*), Pericarpium Citri Reticulatae (*Chen Pi*), Sclerotium Poriae Cocos (*Fu Ling*), Radix Scutellariae Baicalensis (*Huang Qin*), and Rhizoma Coptidis Chinensis (*Huang Lian*) which were boiled into a thick decoction and (taken) with Succus Bambusae (*Zhu Li*) and Succus Zingiberis (*Jiang Zhi*) put in. More than 10 days passed with no effect. Everyone grumbled that the prescription was ill-conceived. I palpated his pulse and realized that his vacuity was yet to be overcome and his phlegm was yet to be led out. Then the same formula continued but with Succus Viticis Negundo (*Jing Li*) added. In another 10 days he was at ease.

One day, my brother-in-law Sui, overeating and drunk, uttered nonsense, raving frenetically with confused vision. The result of questioning (him) was that his dead brother had attached to his body. Everything he said about his brother when alive was true to fact. His uncle who was beside him scolded him, saying that it had nothing to do with ghosts but was simply because he had taken in too much fish and had drunk too much wine. (Thus) it was a trouble caused by phlegm. A big bowl of salt water was poured down his throat which made him vomit one or two *sheng* of phlegm. As a result, a massive sweating broke out. After a night of heavy sleep, he was at ease.

Again, a woman surnamed Jin was in the prime of her life. In a summer month, after she returned from a banquet, her sister-in-law enquired about her *faux pas* of taking the wrong seat. She felt very much ashamed (over this) and subsequently fell ill. She uttered nonsense which was punctuated by the sentence, "It is my humble self to blame." Her pulse was rapid and wiry on both sides. I argued that it was an illness rather than obsession by a (ghost) evil and that if only the spleen were to be supplemented, heat cleared, and phlegm conducted, she would surely recover in a few days. However, her family did not believe me and invited several witches to spray water (on her) and chant incantations. A little more than 10 days later, she died.

Some may ask, "If this disease were not one of (ghost) evil to be treated as a (ghost) evil, how could it have led to death so quickly?" My answer is that, in going to (and from) a banquet in a summer month, the external environment was steaming hot, and, with (her eating) agreeable hot and pungent (food, her) internal environment was (full of) depressive heat. What was worse, (she) had had accumulated phlegm in the past in addition to shame and oppression. (Under such a condition,) her phlegm and heat were untold. Now frightened by the witchery wand, her spirit was frightened and (consequently) her blood became disquieted. Spraying her body with witch water compacted (it) and contracted her skin so that sweat had no way to drain out. With sweat not draining out, steaming heat burned in the internal, and when blood was disquieted, yin was dispersed and yang was unable to stand by itself. How could the result be other than death?

Some may ask, "There is a branch of medicine called supplication[39] in the *Wai Tai Mi Yao (The Secret Essentials of the External Platform).*[40] Is (this branch of medicine) to be repudiated?" My answer is that essence transmission and qi alteration is a small art that can treat minor disorders. If vacuity evils exist in the internal and repletion evils in the external, decent and conventional methods should be used. There are set prescriptions which are quite illuminating and of easy access. Charmed water (can) only (treat) hot phlegm above the diaphragm. After cool water is drunk and meets with stomach heat, (stomach heat) will be cleared and relieved. This indeed may achieve recovery. In case of internal damage with vacuity or in severe winter cold, after charmed water is swallowed down, the stomach will surely be frozen and damaged. Depressive heat existing above and heat evils existing in the exterior require resolving through diaphoresis. If met with cold abruptly, the skin and interstices will become closely sealed. Then from whence can heat be resolved? It will invariably be led to attack inward. (Thus) yin and yang are separated and scattered, and qi and blood are at odds and in conflict. (At that point,) death is close by.

---

[39]   This refers to the fact that in ancient China there was a recognized medical department whose practitioners were essentially shamans and whose practice consisted of incantations, charms, and magic rituals.

[40]   This is a medical book compiled by Wang Tao in 752 CE in 40 volumes. It covered many various branches of medicine and more than 6,000 formulas. External Platform refers to a governmental office which Wang Tao once held. Usually it was the prefecture of a county held by one who had worked in the cabinet. Therefore, this title is sometimes glossed as *Medical Secrets of an Official.*

Treatise on the Face & Nose
Blackened Once Exposed to Cold

All the yang gathers in the head, and the face is yang within yang. In its center is the nose from whose root the *yang ming* begins. All the blood from the whole body is transported to the face and nose, and when it arrives in these yang regions, it becomes most clear and essential blood. Wine tends to flow and is inclined by nature to ascend. It contains great heat and drastic toxins. In heavy drinkers, wine qi fumes and steams their faces and noses. When receiving wine, blood becomes extremely hot. When subjected to cold, hot blood is gathered by yin qi, becoming static, turbid, congealed, and bound. Stagnated and stopped from flowing, (blood) necessarily first turns purple and then black.

(For this condition,) it is necessary to transform static blood in order to free its flow and to enrich and generate new blood in order to enable it to transport and transform. Only thus is the disease cured. My prescription is wine-processed *Si Wu Tang* (Four Materials Decoction) plus stir-fried Radix Scutellariae Baicalensis (*Pian [Qin]*), Sclerotium Poriae Cocos (*Fu Ling*), Pericarpium Citri Reticulatae (*Chen Pi*), raw Radix Glycyrrhizae (*Sheng Gan Cao*), and wine-processed Flos Carthami Tinctorii (*Hong Hua*). Boil with raw Rhizoma Zingiberis (*Sheng Jiang*), brew with powdered Feces Trogopterori Seu Pteromi (*Wu Ling Zhi*), and drink. For those with weak qi, add wine-processed Radix Astragali Membranacei (*Huang Qi*). This never fails to achieve a response.

Treatise on Spontaneous Dropping of the Fetus (*i.e.*, Miscarriage)

Not until yang donates and yin transforms does pregnancy with a (viable) fetus develop. If blood and qi are vacuous and impaired and not enough to nourish the constructive, the fetus will drop spontaneously. Or, if taxation and anger damage the emotions, internal fire may be stirred. This is also capable of (causing) the fetus to drop. In tracing the root and origin (of miscarriage), all (cases) are due to heat. Fire is capable of dispersing things and (also) of creating and transforming (things) in nature. The *Bing Yuan (Origins of Disease)*[41] says that it is wind cold hurting the fetal viscus that causes it to drop. (But) this is not how this disease occurs.

I once saw a woman surnamed Jia who had invariably miscarried around the third month of pregnancy. I felt her pulse which was large and weak on the left hand and choppy when pressure was applied. I realized that she was short of blood. Because (she) was at a wonderful age, it was only (necessary) to supplement (her) central qi in order for the blood to build up itself. It happened to be early summer. I told her to boil a thick decoction of Rhizoma Atractylodis Macrocephalae (*Bai Zhu*) and take it with one *qian* of powdered Radix Scutellariae Baicalensis (*Huang Qin Mo*). After

---

41 This is an abbreviation for the *Zhu Bing Yuan Hou Lun (Treatise on the Origins & Symptoms of Disease)*, the earliest Chinese book which systematically discusses the etiology and symptomatology of disease. It was compiled by Chao Yuan-fang *et al.* in 610 CE.

administration of 30-40 doses, (the child) was secured and delivered safely.

This (case) has led me to the conclusion that, in most cases, miscarriage is justifiably due to internal heat and vacuity. (And,) when speaking of heat and vacuity, it is necessary to (further) divide these in terms of lightness and severity. Practitioners (who) love (their patients') lives are wished not to overlook this.

Treatise on Difficult Delivery

Difficult delivery is commonly seen only in those with depression and oppression as well as the leisured in rich and noble families that are well attended. It never happens to the poor, humble, and toiling. (Current) books of formulas only provide one approach, (using) *Shou Tai Yin* (Thin the Fetus Drink). This formula was designed for Princess Hu Yang.[42] (However,) it affords a far from perfect theory. Why is this? This is because, despite having this formula, (delivery) may be no easier than before.

A clan cousin of mine who was beset by (the past experience of) a difficult delivery had chosen to abort each time she conceived (rather than experience another difficult delivery). I took great pity on her. Seeing that she was fat in form and labored at sewing and knitting, (I) had mused (on her case)

---

42   This refers to the sister of Liu Che (156-87 BCE), Emperor Wu of the Han dynasty.

for 10 days when I suddenly realized that her (condition) was just opposite to that of Princess Hu Yang who was well attended, who certainly had replete qi, and whose qi could be made peaceful and calm by consumption so that she would have easy delivery. (However, because of this cousin's) fat form I realized (she) had qi vacuity and (because of her) sitting for long (periods) I realized (her) qi did not circulate. (Further, this prolonged sitting then) made (her) qi even weaker. Thus prolonged sitting and the fat form of the mother caused the fetus (in the uterus) to be unable to move itself. (Therefore,) it was necessary to supplement the mother's qi and then the child might become strong and easily delivered. At that time, she was in her fifth or sixth month of pregnancy. (I) prescribed her more than 10 doses of *Zi Su Yin* (Perilla Drink) from the *Da Quan Fang (Complete Collection of Formulas)*[43] with certain qi-supplementing medicinals added. This resulted in her getting a (baby) boy without a hitch in labor. (I) have since prescribed this formula with additions and subtractions in accordance with the mothers' form, color, and character and with reference to the seasons, and none of the takers have failed to respond well. Based on this, (I) have named this formula *Da Da Sheng San* (Major Expedite Delivery Powder).

---

[43] *I.e.*, the *Fu Ren Da Quan Liang Fang (Complete Collection of Fine Formulas for Women)* compiled by Chen Zi-ming (circa 1190-1272 CE). Also known as Chen Liang-fu, he was a native of Lin Chau now called Fuzhou, Jiangxi Province. He is also the author of *Wai Ke Jing Yao (The Essence & Essentials of External [Medicine])*.

Treatise on Dribbling (Urination) Due to the Bladder Having Been Damaged During Difficult Delivery

Cases are often seen where, because of the carelessness of the midwife, the urinary bladder is broken and injured so that strangury disease arises. This may develop into a disabling disease.

One day, a lady named Xu contracted such a disease while of robust age. I thought that since broken and wounded muscles in the external can be completely mended, the bladder, though inside the abdomen, might also well be treated. Then I felt her pulse which was extremely vacuous. As it is said, "The cause of difficult delivery is usually qi vacuity, and following difficult delivery, the blood and qi are the more vacuous." (I, therefore,) tried drastically supplementing (blood and qi) with Radix Panacis Ginseng (*Ren Shen*) and Rhizoma Atractylodis Macrocephalae (*Bai Zhu*) as sovereigns, Rhizoma Ligustici Wallichii (*Chuan Xiong*) and Radix Angelicae Sinensis (*Dang Gui*) as ministers, and Semen Pruni Persicae (*Tao Ren*), Pericarpium Citri Reticulatae (*Chen Pi*), Radix Astragali Membranacei (*Huang Qi*), and Sclerotium Poriae Cocos (*Fu Ling*) as assistants. These were boiled in a soup of pig (or) sheep's bladder and drunk when extremely hungry. Each dose was prescribed at one *liang*. After a month, (the patient) was at ease. Perhaps, because the blood and qi grew sharply, the bladder recovered by itself. (I am) afraid, with (even) a little delay, success would have been hardly possible.

Treatise on Deviated Uterus Disease in Pregnant Women

Deviated uterus (*i. e.*, fetal pressure) disease often occurs to pregnant women who are weak, who (experience) excessive depression and oppression, who are quick tempered and have an impatient disposition, and who eat a thick flavored (diet). The ancient formulas (for this condition) are all composed of lubricating and disinhibiting, coursing and abducting medicinals. Rarely do they correspond (to the patient's pattern) or are (therefore) efficacious. This leads me to think that when the uterus, dragged (downward) by the fetus, is turned to one side, its ligation becomes entangled and thus (the uterus) is blocked. (Thus) if the fetus were to be lifted and suspended in the center, the uterine ligation would be coursed and the water passageways naturally disinhibited. However, the sagging of any fetus invariably has some reason.

One day, the concubine of the Wu's household suffered from this disease. (I) felt her pulse which was somewhat choppy on both hands and wiry when pressure was applied. However, it was less inharmonious on the left hand. I said that this (disease) had been contracted as a result of worry and anxiety. A choppy (pulse) indicated scant blood but abundant qi. A wiry (pulse) indicated the existence of rheum. With scant blood, the uterus was weak, unable to uplift itself, while with abundant qi and the existence of rheum, the middle burner was unclear and spilling (over). Thus the uterus had to get out of the way, tending to go downward and, therefore, sagged. (I) prescribed *Si Wu Tang* (Four Materials Decoction) plus Radix Panacis Ginseng (*Ren Shen*),

Rhizoma Atractylodis Macrocephalae (*Bai Zhu*), Rhizoma Pinelliae Ternatae (*Ban Xia*), Pericarpium Citri Reticulatae (*Chen Pi*), raw Radix Glycyrrhizae (*Sheng Gan Cao*), and raw Rhizoma Zingiberis (*Sheng Jiang*). These were (boiled and) taken on an empty stomach. Thereupon, her throat was probed with fingers to (induce) vomiting of the decoction. A little while later, when her qi calmed down, another dose was administered. The same (maneuver was performed) once again the next morning. Eight doses were administered in this way and (the patient) was at ease. (Afterwards, I) was not certain whether this method was a good one or not and was afraid that it was but a chance hit. Later, I tried it on several more persons, achieving effect (in those cases) as well. (However, this method's) conclusive results remain to be further proved.

(Zhang) Zhong-jing said: "When a woman who used to be fat and exuberant in the past with fullness all over the body becomes markedly emaciated with emptiness and reduction all over the body, the uterine ligation is entangled and there is shifting of the uterus." The meaning (of this saying) is obscure, but there should be someone able to understand it.

Treatise on Hardness of the Breasts

The breasts are where the *yang ming* channel passes, and the nipples are where the *jue yin* homes. (Some) breast-feeding mothers do not know how to regulate and nurture (themselves). As a result of counterflow due to anger and indignation, obstruction caused by depression and oppression and the brewing of thick flavors, the qi of the *jue yin* is stopped from circulating. Consequently, the portals are blocked and milk cannot exit. (Then) the blood of the *yang ming* boils. It becomes so hot, it transforms into pus. There are also cases where the suckling baby has stagnated phlegm around the diaphragm with the mouth qi burning hot. They may sleep with the nipple held in (their) mouth. Blown by (this) hot qi, (the mother's) nipple grows a tubercle.

At the outset, (one) must, in defiance of the pain, soften (the nodes) by rubbing and suck the breast milk all out. Then (the nodes) will be dispersed and dissipated. If one misses the chance to treat (this condition at an early stage), *yong* and boils are bound to develop. The treatment method is to dredge stasis from the *jue yin* with Pericarpium Viridis Citri Reticulatae (*Qing Pi*), to clear heat from the *yang ming* with finely ground Gypsum (*Shi Gao*), to move away static, turbid blood with raw Nodus Radicis Glycyrrhizae (*Sheng Gan Cao Jie*), and to disperse swelling and conduct toxins with Semen Trichosanthis Kirlowii (*Gua Lou Zi*). Myrrha (*Mo Yao*), green (*i.e.*, fresh) Folium Citri (*Qing Ju Ye*), Spina Gleditschiae Sinensis (*Zao Jiao Ci*), Flos Lonicerae Japonicae (*Jin Yin Hua*), and Radix Angelicae Sinensis (*Dang Gui*) may be added. (This formula) can be taken either in the form of a powder or a decoction, allowing for additions and subtractions at (one's) discretion. However, a small amount of wine should be used as an assistant. If two to three cones of Folium Artemisiae Argyii (*Ai*) are moxaed at the place that is swollen, the effect will be more rapid.

Those vulgar (*i. e.*, common or mediocre) practitioners who take pleasure in parading (around) tend to unscrupulously perform needling or lancing, thus causing unnecessary pain (in the patient). This is truly lamentable and regrettable.

If (a woman) is out of favor with (her) husband or (her)

brother- or sister-in-law, worry and anger, depression and oppression will accumulate day and night. The spleen qi will be dispersed and impeded and the liver qi will counterflow wildly. As a result, a dormant node will develop gradually as big as a chess piece with no pain or itching. It takes tens of years to develop into a sunken sore, called suckling breast rock because it forms a depression like a rock cave. (This) is (then) incurable. If, at the initial stage of its generation, (one) eliminates the root of the disease by keeping the heart tranquil and the spirit calm and then carries out a (proper) treatment method, there is the possibility of healing.

The wife of my clan nephew contracted this pattern at the age of 18. Her form and pulse were found a little replete, but she was of quick and impatient temper. The married pair were on amicable terms. It was her half-blood sister-in-law who caused the difficulty. (I) administered a simple formula, *Qing Pi Tang* (Green Orange Peel Decoction) and, from time to time, *Si Wu Tang* (Four Materials Decoction) with additions and subtractions (plus) medicinals for moving the channels and connecting vessels. Two months later, (she) was at ease.

Treatise on Gestation

It was Chu Cheng's[44] theory that the fetus becomes either a male or a female due to the essence or blood (coming) after

---

[44] Chu Cheng was the author of the *Chu Shi Yi Shu (Master Chu's Posthumous Book)* compiled during the Southern Qi dynasty (479-502 CE). This book discusses many interesting aspects of physiology and pathology.

or before. But as for my dull self, (I) am keenly skeptical about this. Later, I read a book by Li Dong-yuan in which it is explained that one or two days after the termination of the menses, when the sea of blood has just become clear and essence is overwhelming the blood, that which reacts forms into a male, while four or five days later, when the blood vessels are already effulgent and essence is not overwhelming blood any longer, that which reacts forms into a female. This is a convincing theory.

The *Yi* (*[Classic of] Change*) says: "*Qian* (*i.e.*, heavenly) *dao* forms the male, while *kun* (*i.e.*, earthly) *dao* forms the female." *Qian* and *kun* are the dispositions and natures of yin and yang. Left and right are the roads of yin and yang. (And) male and female are the bearing and image of yin and yang. The essence of the father and the blood of the mother react upon one another so as to meet. (In this process,) essence is the donor. Blood containing and developing this into a seed (or child), thus are the ten thousand things bred and inaugurated by the *qian* (*i.e.*, heavenly) source. Blood forming the wrapper (of the seed), thus are the ten thousand things bred and generated by the *kun* (*i.e.*, earthly) source. When yin and yang mate, a fetus is coagulated, and the place where it hides is called the child's palace. This has a ligation below and two branches above, one reaching the left and the other reaching the right. If essence overwhelms blood, yang becomes the ruler. It receives qi from the left (branch of the) child's palace and a male takes shape. If essence is unable to overwhelm blood, yin becomes the ruler. It receives qi from the right (branch of the) child's palace, and a female takes shape.

Some may ask, "I know how to differentiate male and female. (However, some) males cannot be fathers; (some) females cannot be mothers; and (still others) have the dual form of (both) male and female. How then can one differentiate these?" My answer is that a male who cannot be a father is one who has received inadequate yang qi; that a female who cannot be a mother is one who has been obstructed in receiving yin qi; and that one with a dual form is a product of yin invaded by variegated (*i.e.*, mixed and disorderly) qi. (Of the last kind), there are various different types. There are two types of femininity embracing masculinity. One can become a wife when met with a male, but a husband when met with a female. The other is capable of being a wife but not a husband. In addition, there is (a type of) femininity embracing all masculinity. This is an extreme case of variegation.

Some may ask, "Invasion of variegated qi is seen solely in the yin, but why is there such a difference in the form (produced) by (this) invasion?" My answer is that a yin body is vacuous, so it is easily invaded by (such) variegated qi. (Once) invaded by variegated qi, yin and yang are blended, no one ruling over the other. (Thus the fetus) pertains neither to the left nor the right. It receives qi from between the two branches and takes (its) shape depending on the lightness or heaviness (*i.e.*, the severity) of the variegated qi received. Therefore, dual forms cannot always be the same.

Treatise on the *Ren Ying* & *Qi Kou*

The six yang and six yin pulses belong respectively to the left and right hands. (The pulses of) the heart, small intestine, liver, gallbladder, kidneys, and urinary bladder are located on the left which governs the blood. (The pulses of) the lungs, large intestine, spleen, stomach, life gate, and triple burner are located on the right which governs qi. A male results from qi turning into the fetus and, therefore, is governed by qi. A female results from blood turning into the fetus and, therefore, is governed by blood. In a male with an enduring disease, if the *qi kou*[45] (pulse) is fuller than the *ren ying*[46] (pulse), there is (still) stomach qi and the disease, even though (otherwise) serious, is curable. In a female with an enduring disease, if the *ren ying* is fuller than the *qi kou*, there is (still) stomach qi and the disease, even though (otherwise) serious, is curable. (Pulses) contrary to this are counterflow (*i.e.*, unfavorable).

Some may ask, "The *ren ying* is located on the left (hand), while the *qi kou* (is located) on the right. Their locations are the same in males and females and are unchanging. It is said in the *Mai Fa Zan (The Pulse in Verse)*[47]: 'A left large (pulse) is favorable in men, while a right large (pulse) is favorable in women.' Why is your explanation opposite?" (My) answer is that, in the *Mai Jing (Pulse Classic)*[48], Wang Shu-he tirelessly

---

[45] *Qi kou* means qi opening or qi mouth. Here the qi opening refers specifically to the pulse in the *cun* or inch position on the right hand rather than to the arterial pulse at the styloid process of the wrist as a whole.

[46] *Ren ying* means human prognosis. Here it refers to the pulse in the *cun* position on the left hand and not to the pulse at the acupuncture point on the front of the neck of the same name.

[47] The *Mai Fa Zan* mentioned here may be an ancient classic on pulse examination which is mentioned in the *Nei Jing* as the *Mai Jing*, but, if so, it is long lost.

[48] This is the earliest extant and most important Chinese book devoted to the pulse written by Wang Shu-he (circa 210-285 CE). Wang Shu-he, also known as Wang Xi, was the editor who separated Zhang Zhong-jing's work into what is now known as the *Shang Han Lun* and *Jin Gui Yao Lue*.

taught physicians that the left and right hand are referred to with the (attending) physician's (hands) as the standard. If the patient's (hands) were taken as the standard, it would be a gross blunder, no less than a deviation of a thousand *li*!

Treatise on Spring Diffusion

(The character) spring (implies) agitation to get going. (In spring,) yang qi is ascending and floating, while grass and trees are sprouting. (Thus everything is) agitating to get going and to move. The sages in the past have said that, in spring, the human qi is in the head and disease, if any, should be treated by ejection. It is also stated that the great method for cold damage stipulates that, in the spring, it is appropriate to employ ejection. Diffusing is spoken of as upraising, suggesting the method of ejection through the above.

Nowadays, lay and vulgar persons assume that sores, diaphragmatic fullness, and worm (*i.e.*, parasite) accumulations are impossible to cure if not treated in spring by diffusion and catharsis with toxic medicinals. It follows that physicians tend to prescribe Semen Pharbitidis (*Qian Niu*), Semen Crotonis (*Ba Dou*), Radix Et Rhizoma Rhei (*Da Huang*), Fructus Citri Seu Ponciri (*Zhi Qiao*), and Radix Ledebouriellae Sesloidis (*Fang Feng*) in the shape of pills. These are called *Chun Xuan Wan* (Spring Diffusing Pills. They) are administered in the second and third months. When the bowels are loosened, they are stopped. When diarrhea is first brought on, the viscera and bowels are freed and there is temporary relief. (People) do not understand that when qi is ascending above, the yin below is extremely weak. If disinhibiting medicinals (*i.e.*, laxatives) are used to mutilate and rob yin, the harm is untold. Moreover, (Zhang) Zhong-jing never employed precipitating formulas, such as *Cheng Qi Tang* (Support the Qi Decoction) unless there was great fullness, great solid hardness, dry stools with passing flatulence, pressure in the rectum below, and absence of exterior signs. Otherwise, (he) did not use this method (of precipitation). If all the signs indicating precipitation are not present, it is yet (even more) necessary to suspend it and wait. Cathartics and disinhibitors absolutely cannot be used without warrant.

My late uncle, who was of fat form but thin skeleton, fed (habitually) on thick flavors. He had a reflective character (but) was credulous enough to believe some hearsay at the age of 50. In the middle of the third month (of that year, he) bought a packet of *Chun Xuan Wan*. After taking it, two to three bowel movements were induced. (From then on,) every year he took (a packet) as a rule. At 53 years old, early in the seventh month when (the weather) was extremely hot, (he) died a death from no disease. Is this not a disaster resulting from the unjustified assumption that diffusing in spring means catharsis in spring?

Calling forth the lower through the upper is called diffusion. It is clear that the word diffusion means ejection. Master Zhang Zi-he gave a detailed discussion about this. Could the past sage have made his statement unscrupulously? (He) must undoubtedly have reviewed and checked it very carefully. After (the death of my uncle,) there were several more deaths (from the same medication). For that reason, my dull self is setting this down to show people of later generations as a warning.

Treatise on Mellow Wine Being Fit to Drink Cold

Mellow wine has the nature of great heat and great toxicity. Of delicate fragrance and nice flavor, it is a treat to the mouth. (It) is able to move qi and harmonize blood. It is also good for the body. Therefore, drinkers are tempted to drink more than (what is) good (for them) without being aware, forgetting that the lungs are ascribed to metal which is in awe of fire by nature. The lungs, whose bodies are fragile and which are located high, are the governor of qi, mother of the kidneys, and husband[49] of wood. When wine goes down the throat and diaphragm, the lungs are the first to receive it.

Wine, if mellow, is justifiably fit to drink cold. It passes by the lungs and enters the stomach. Then (it) gradually warms the lungs. First (the lungs) gain the cold within the warmth which is able to supplement qi. This is the first benefit. Then (the stomach) gains the warmth within the cold which is able to nurture the stomach. This is the second benefit. Cold wine, slow in moving, is transported and transformed gradually, (so) it is impossible to drink ravenously. This is the third benefit. Ancient people never drank more than three *jue*[50] in a day even (when pressed) with a hundred prostrations, so

---

[49] That which restrains is called the husband according to five phase theory.

[50] This is an ancient wine vessel with three legs and a loop handle.

70

that they were free from both wine disease and wine disaster.

Recently, I consulted the *Li Jing (The Classic of Rites)*[51] which says: "Drinking should look for the winter time." Here drinking refers to wine (and) looking for means assimilating. Winter time implies cold. (I have also) referred to the *Nei Jing* which says that heat causes one to make use of cold. What a profound meaning! (But) now things are different. People disregard (the risk of) injury and only seek for entertainment. Drinking heated (wine) consists in three pleasures. Diaphragmatic stagnation is freed and relieved. The tongue and throat (are stimulated by) acridity and feel comfortable. (And) drinking quantities is (thus) made possible. What is forgotten is that, since wine tends to ascend by nature, qi invariably follows it (upward). Phlegm is depressed above and urination becomes inhibited below. Since the lungs are subjected to thieving evils, the body of metal must be dried.

When cold and cool (beverages) are drunk in great quantities, heat is depressed in the internal. When lung qi receives heat, it must be greatly damaged and consumed. At the initial stage, the disease is shallow, perhaps consisting of vomiting, possibly spontaneous sweating, possibly sores, possibly drinker's nose, possibly loosed bowels, or possibly heart and spleen pain. (At this stage,) it is not yet impossible to remove (this heat) through effusing and dissipating. (However,) if it lasts for a long (time), the disease will be deeper, giving rise to wasting thirst, thirst, internal jaundice, lung atony, internal hemorrhoids, drum distention, and loss of eyesight or wheezing dyspnea, taxation cough, and epilepsy. It also can be a disease difficult to identify. Unless under a good eye, it

---

[51] Also named the *Li Ji (Records of Rites)*, this book is one of the so-called Five Classics of Confucianism.

is not easy to handle and treat. How can one not be cautious?.

Some may say, "There is a popular saying that one cup of cold wine requires two cups of blood to move it, which makes it clear that wine is unfit to be drunk cold." I should say that those are the words of barbarians. Now, with reference to the classics and appealing to reasons, (I) present the (above) as admonition.

Treatise on the Necessity of Differentiating *Yong* & *Ju* in Accordance with Channels & Connecting Vessels

Of the six yang channels and six yin channels which spread and distribute all over the body, some are abundant in qi but scanty in blood, some are scanty in qi but abundant in blood, (and) some are abundant both in qi and blood. (Therefore,) they can not be dealt with (all) in one way. (*Yong* and *ju* may grow at) the vital places and the places near to the vacuous, tender, and thin parts. This has already been touched on by the past sages. Only an approach to their division in accordance with the channels has never (yet) been heard. What is this (approach)?

Because they are abundant in qi but scanty in blood, only *yong* and *ju* that are generated by the *shao yang* and *jue yin* out of all the channels justifiably need (particular) prevention. Originally, their blood is scant, and the muscles and flesh (associated with them) have difficulty growing. (Therefore,) if sores do not heal for a long time, they will inevitably develop into a fatal pattern. If one does not take into consideration the original deficiency of blood in those channels and recklessly employs toxin-dispelling disinhibitors so that the blood of the yin phase is felled, disaster will follow upon the heels (of the treatment). Please let (me) give a report of a couple of successes and failures (in the treatment of such lesions) as a lesson for those who will come later.

At nearly 50 years of age, an uncle of mine who worried his entire life (and) had a weak physique and spirit taxation suddenly grew a small, red swelling the size of a chestnut on the outer (*i.e.*, lateral) portion of (his) left upper arm.[52] Seeing this, I told him not to overlook it and prescribed for him a decoction of unprocessed Radix Panacis Ginseng (*Ren Shen*) in large dosage, preferably two to three *jin* (administered all at one time). Not believing (me), he arbitrarily took several doses in small amounts (but) stopped the administration before a resolution (was affected). A little more than 10 days later, when there happened to be a wind so strong as to pull up trees, a red line appeared on the sore. (This line) turned across the scapula on the back and extended straight to the ribs on the right. I said that there was no other choice but to administer Radix Panacis Ginseng in large quantities plus small amounts of supplementing medicinals such as Radix Angelicae Sinensis (*Dang Gui*), Rhizoma Ligustici Wallichii (*Chuan Xiong*), Pericarpium Citri Reticulatae (*Chen Pi*), and Rhizoma Atractylodis Macrocephalae (*Bai Zhu*). Then (I) prescribed this formula for two months and (the patient) was at ease.

Another (case involved) Li, a friend in Dong Yang, who was over 30 years of age. (He had) a thin form and thick skin.

---

[52] This area belongs to the triple burner channel of the hand *shao yang*.

Because he had suffered from worry and frustration in succession, and, moreover, because of toiling in addition to overindulgence in beauty's charms, he abruptly had a red swelling the size of a chestnut growing on the outer side of (his) left leg.[53] A physician, after making certain that his great bowel[54] was strong and solid, prescribed him two doses of *Cheng Qi* (Support the Qi [Decoction]) in order to precipitate but with no effect. Another physician instructed (him) to administer Radix Et Rhizoma Rhei (*Da Huang*), Cinnabaris (*Zhu Sha*), debarked Radix Glycyrrhizae (*Sheng Fen Cao*), and Sanguis Draconis (*Qi Lin Jie*). Two to three doses were taken in addition (to the preceding formula). Half a month later, I was called for an inspection. (I had to) say the case was done for.

Another friend named Li, aged over 40, (had) a whitish facial complexion and severely taxed spirit. (He) suddenly grew a red swelling the size of a peach in (his) lateral costal region. A physician instructed (him) to use a *Shen* formula[55] but (this) was laughed at and rejected. Then *Liu Qi Yin* (Flow the

---

[53]   This area belongs to the gallbladder channel of the foot *shao yang*.

[54]   The stomach is often referred to as the great bowel or *da fu* in Chinese medicine. However, here it refers to bound stools. These are then impugned to a dry large intestine.

[55]   There are tens of formulas which begin with the word *shen* (spirit, god, miraculous, etc.) which are indicated for this kind of disease. The translator, however, suspects that here it refers merely to a decoction made of Radix Panacis Ginseng (*Ren Shen*). Such decoction is often referred to as *Shen Cao* (Miraculous or Divine Grass).

Qi Drink)[56] and *Shi Xuan San* (Ten Diffusion Powder)[57] were administered higgledy-piggledy. A little more than 10 days later I was sent for an inspection. I said that, since not only had he been denied supplementing medicinals but had been administered many resolving and disinhibiting medicinals, both his qi and blood were exhausted. Afterwards, (my words) proved true.

Some may ask, "Isn't the *tai yang* channel abundant in blood and scanty in qi? Then why is the growth of *ju* on the buttocks, which at first (causes) no severe bitterness (*i.e.*, suffering), often irretrievable? Can your honor offer a treatment for it?" My answer is that the buttocks are located behind and below the lower abdomen, this being yin within yin. There is a long way to it and its location is remote.

---

[56] This is composed of Pericarpium Arecae (*Da Fu Pi*), 1 *qian*, Pericarpium Citri Reticulatae (*Chen Pi*), Sclerotium Rubrum Poriae Cocos (*Chi Fu Ling*), Radix Angelicae Sinensis (*Dang Gui*), Radix Albus Paeoniae Lactiflorae (*Bai Shao*), Rhizoma Ligustici Wallichii (*Chuan Xiong*), Radix Astragali Membranacei (*Huang Qi*), Rhizoma Pinelliae Ternatae (*Ban Xia*), Fructus Immaturus Citri Seu Ponciri (*Zhi Shi*), Radix Glycyrrhizae (*Gan Cao*), and Radix Ledebouriellae Sesloidis (*Fang Feng*), 7.5 *fen* for each of the above, Folium Perillae Frutescentis (*Su Ye*), Radix Linderae Strychnifoliae (*Wu Yao*), Pericarpium Viridis Citri Reticulatae (*Qing Pi*), and Radix Platycodi Grandiflori (*Jie Geng*), 1.5 *qian* for each of the above, Radix Saussureae Seu Vladimiriae (*Mu Xiang*), 2.5 *fen*, 3 slices of Rhizoma Zingiberis (*Jiang*), and 2 pieces of Fructus Zizyphi Jujubae (*Zao*).

[57] This consists of Radix Astragali Membranacei (*Huang Qi*), Radix Angelicae Sinensis (*Dang Gui*), and Radix Panacis Ginseng (*Ren Shen*), 2 *qian* for each of the above, Cortex Magnoliae Officinalis (*Hou Po*), Radix Platycodi Grandiflori (*Jie Geng*), Rhizoma Ligustici Wallichii (*Chuan Xiong*), Radix Ledebouriellae Sesloidis (*Fang Feng*), Radix Glycyrrhizae (*Gan Cao*), and Radix Angelicae (*Bai Zhi*), 1 *qian* for each of the above, and Cortex Cinnamomi (*Gui Xin*), 3 *fen*.

Although (the *tai yang*) is said to be abundant in blood, qi is not transported there (in quantity). Since qi is inhibited, blood rarely goes there. After middle age, (one should take care) not to grow *yong*. As soon as there arises a pain (or) swelling, the pulses and signs should be examined, and once vacuity weakness is observed, enriching and supplementing (medicinals) should be administered. If there is no depletion of blood and qi, a happy end will be ensured. If (one) uses conventional medications to dispel heat, remove toxins, and relax the qi, the disaster of evacuating vacuity would be laid fingers on (*i.e.*, would be close by and obviously evident).

Treatise on *Pi Yue Wan* (Spleen Constraint Pills)[58]

Cheng Wu-ji[59] says:

To constrain means to bind and restrain. If the stomach is strong but the spleen is weak, humors and fluids are

---

[58] This is composed of Semen Cannabis Sativae (*Ma Ren*), 2 *sheng*, Radix Paeoniae Lactiflorae (*Shao Yao*), 0.5 *jin*, stir-fried Fructus Immaturus Citri Seu Ponciri (*Zhi Shi*), 0.5 *jin*, Radix Et Rhizoma Rhei (*Da Huang*), 1 *jin*, stir-fried Cortex Magnoliae Officinalis (*Hou Po*), 1 *chi* (*i.e.*, 1/3 meter), and parched Semen Pruni Armeniacae (*Xing Ren*), 1 *sheng*. The above are powdered and made into pills with honey.

[59] Cheng Wu-ji (1062-1155 CE) was a preeminent physician in the late Song dynasty whose masterpiece is *Zhu Jie Shang Han Lun* (*An Annotated Treatise on Cold Damage*). It is the earliest Chinese commentary on Zhang Zhong-jing's *Shang Han Lun* (*Treatise on Cold Damage*).

restrained from spreading in every direction but are transported to the urinary bladder. As a result, urine is voided frequently and stools become hard. Therefore, (this condition) is called constrained spleen.

These pills (*i.e.*, *Pi Yue Wan*) are administered to precipitate the bound dryness of the spleen. Thus the intestines are moistened and the bind is transformed, while the fluid flows into the stomach. (Therefore,) defecation is disinhibited and urine is voided infrequently, resulting in recuperation. My dull self (however,) has a keen doubt about this.

What is (this doubt)? Since it is said to be constrained, the spleen (must) be too weak to transport. With a weak spleen, earth is deficient. This must be because the spleen qi is dispersed and spleen blood is consumed. If the original cause is traced, following great precipitation and great diaphoresis in (treating) chronic disease, yin blood becomes dried and desiccated and internal fire burns vehemently. (This) heat damages the original qi and further (damages) the spleen, thus giving rise to this pattern. Damaging the original qi means that, since lung metal is subjected to fire, there is nothing to contain qi. Damaging the spleen means that, when the lungs, the son of the spleen, are consumed, fluids are exhausted and (the lungs) have to steal (their) mother's qi to rescue themselves. When metal is consumed, wood has little in awe (of other viscera), and, much as earth intends to, it is impossible to escape from injury. When the spleen fails to exercise its duty of transportation and conveyance and the lungs lose their office of transportation and delivery, the stools reasonably become constipated and are difficult to evacuate. Whereas urine is voided frequently without being stored and gathered. (For this condition), it is only reasonable to enrich and nurture yin blood so that the fire of solitary yang should not glow and metal should be enabled to exercise clearing and transformation. (Then) wood evil is no longer unable to be restrained and spleen earth becomes clear and strong enough to transport and move. Only thus is it possible for essence and fluids to enter the stomach and are the intestines moistened and unblocked.

Now (for this condition,) use Radix Et Rhizoma Rhei (*Da Huang*) as the sovereign and Fructus Immaturus Citri Seu Ponciri (*Zhi Shi*) and Cortex Magnoliae Officinalis (*Hou Po*) as the ministers. Although used as assistants and envoys, Radix Paeoniae Lactiflorae (*Shao Yao*) enriches blood and Semen Cannabis Sativae (*Ma Ren*) and Semen Pruni Armeniacae (*Xing Ren*) moisten with warmth. (This formula) never fails to affect recovery even when employed in case of extreme heat and replete qi.

(However,) my dull self has a fear that only in the West and the North, where the earth qi is high and thick, and the people have strong and sturdy physique, can (this formula) be put to use. If it is applied to the people in the South and the East or to those with blood and qi not replenished despite exuberant heat, though temporary unblocking might be effected, their spleen would become weaker and their intestines drier. Later students who intend to use this formula should know that, in the West and North, opening bind must be made the rule, while in the East and South, the rule is to moisten dryness. Be sure not to tune a *se*[60] with the pegs glued.

---

[60] This is a plucked musical instrument with twenty-five strings, somewhat similar to a zither.

Treatise on Drum Distention

The heart and lungs, which are ascribed to yang, are located above, while the liver and kidneys, which are ascribed to yin, are located below. The spleen, located in the center, which is also yin, is ascribed to earth. The classic (*i.e.*, the *Nei Jing*) states:

> Drink and food enter the stomach which floats essence qi and transports it up to the spleen. (Then) spleen qi spreads the essence which comes up home to the lungs to free and adjust the flow of the water passageways, transporting (water) down to the urinary bladder. Water essence spreads in the four directions and the five channels run side by side.

Thus the spleen gains the tranquil virtue of earth and has the vigor of the movement of heaven. For that reason, it enables the yang of the heart and lungs to descend and the yin of the kidneys and liver to ascend, resulting in the advantageous communication between heaven and earth. Such is (the state) of a healthy person.

The seven affects damage the internal, the six environmental excesses invade from outside, food and drink are had without restraint, and chamber taxation causes vacuity. (Any of these causes may) damage spleen earth yin (and consequently,) the office of transportation and conveyance may fail to carry out its duty. Although the stomach (still) receives grains, (the spleen) cannot transport or transform them. As a result, yang keeps on upbearing itself and yin keeps on downbearing itself, resulting in the disadvantageous divorce between heaven and earth. When this happens, clearness and turbidity are confused together and the tunnels are congested and held up. Qi transforms into the turbid, and blood becomes stagnated with depressive heat (being generated). When heat remains for long, qi transforms into dampness. Dampness and heat mutually engender, thus giving rise to distention and fullness. This is what the classic calls drum distention because, though hard and full, the abdomen (supplementation in the Chinese text [tr.]) is empty with nothing inside, (thus) resembling a drum. The disease is persistent and firmly fixed, (and is, therefore,) difficult to cure. It is also called gu.[61] Because it is as if (one were) invaded and being eaten by worms, therefore, (this kind of distention) is called gu.

In reference to the method of treatment (for this condition), it is justifiably appropriate to supplement the spleen, and it is also necessary to nurture lung metal to restrain wood in order that the spleen is freed from the worry of bandit evils. (One should also) enrich kidney water to restrain fire in order that the lungs are enabled to exercise purification. Abstain from salty flavor lest it should assist the evil and cut off frenetic desire in order to protect the maternal qi. Thus there are none who are not (subsequently) at ease.

(However,) some physicians, unaware that (this) disease originates from vacuity, are eager for a rapid effect to show off their ability and to seek for reward. And patients, bitterly (distressed) by urgent distention, prefer (qi-)moving and disinhibiting medicinals just to seek (some) temporary relief, not knowing that relaxation for a day or a half may only be followed by more serious swelling. The disease evils (then) become more serious, and the true qi is damaged. (In this

---

[61] This is a legendary venomous insect which was believed to enter the body and cause a big-bellied disease.

case,) death is not far off. Of ancient formulas, only *Yu Yu Liang Wan* (Limonite Pills)[62], also named *Shi Zhong Huang Wan* (Inside Stone Yellow Pills) or *Zi Jin Wan* (Purple Gold Pills), restrain the liver and supplement the spleen with an exceptional specific efficacy. However, these, too, should be added to and subtracted from in accordance with the signs and seasons.

My friend, Yu Ren-shu, a Confucian scholar and physician (himself), who had been struck by continual family mishaps, contracted this kind of disease at 50 years of age. He took self-prepared *Yu Yu Liang Wan*. I examined his pulse which was choppy and rapid. (I) said that those pills were newly prepared and still retained the furnace's fire evil and that they contained too many warm and hot medicinals. He should have made additions and subtractions (to the formula). One should not stick to a formula (with no adaptation according to the patient's individual situation). Yu smiled, saying that contemporary people are inferior to the ancients and that this formula allows for no additions or subtractions. After one month's administration, (he) bled at the mouth and nose, became scrawny and emaciated, and then died.

---

[62]   This is composed of Serpent's Bezoar (*i.e.*, pisiform clay iron ore, *She Huang*) and Limonite (*Yu Yu Liang*), 3 *liang* each, and Radix Et Rhizoma Notopterygii (*Qiang Huo*), roasted Radix Saussureae Seu Vladimiriae (*Mu Xiang*), Sclerotium Poriae Cocos (*Fu Ling*), Rhizoma Ligustici Wallichii (*Chuan Xiong*), Radix Achyranthis (*Niu Xi*), baked Fructus Cardamomi (*Bai Dou Kou*), Fructus Foeniculi Vulgaris (*Tu Hui Xiang*), baked Rhizoma Curcumae Zedoariae (*E Zhu*), Cortex Cinnamomi (*Gui Xin*), baked Rhizoma Zingiberis (*Jiang*), Pericarpium Viridis Citri Reticulatae (*Qing Pi*), baked Rhizoma Sparganii (*San Leng*), Fructus Tribuli Terrestris (*Bai Ji Li*), baked Radix Praeparatus Aconiti Carmichaeli (*Fu Zi*), and Radix Angelicae Sinensis (*Dang Gui*), 0.5 *liang* for each of the above.

81

Again, Yang, a friend aged nearly 50, was addicted to wine. Having been diseased with malaria for half a year, (he) contracted the disease of distention. Assuming that he was bound to die, he came over for a treatment. I examined his pulse which was wiry and choppy and large when pressure was applied. His malaria remained to be overcome, and he had thin hands and feet with an enlarged belly like a spider. I instructed (him) to use Radix Panacis Ginseng (*Ren Shen*) and Rhizoma Atractylodis Macrocephalae (*Bai Zhu*) as sovereigns, Radix Angelicae Sinensis (*Dang Gui*), Rhizoma Ligustici Wallichii (*Chuan Xiong*), and Radix Paeoniae Lactiflorae (*Shao Yao*) as ministers, and Rhizoma Coptidis Chinensis (*Huang Lian*), Pericarpium Citri Reticulatae (*Chen Pi*), Sclerotium Poriae Cocos (*Fu Ling*), and Cortex Magnoliae Officinalis (*Hou Po*) as assistants, all of which were to be boiled with a small amount of raw Radix Glycyrrhizae (*Sheng Gan Cao*) into a thick decoction and drunk. He needed to take this three times a day and, in addition, to strictly abide by the prohibitions and commandments. A month later, his malaria was cured following perspiration. Half a year later, his urination became long and the distention was overcome. During (this) course (of treatment, the formula) underwent (various) additions and subtractions in a small way. Throughout, the fundamental objectives remained the supplementation qi and removal dampness.

Again, a Master Chen, aged over 40, was addicted to wine. He occasionally had had blood in (his) stools, and, in the spring, began to suffer from distention with a black complexion and enlarged abdomen. (He) looked like a ghost. I felt his pulse which was rapid and choppy and somewhat weak when pressure was applied. I prescribed *Si Wu Tang* (Four Materials Decoction), adding Rhizoma Coptidis Chinensis (*Huang Lian*), Radix Scutellariae Baicalensis (*Huang Qin*), Caulis Akebiae Mutong (*Mu Tong*), Rhizoma Atractylodis

Macrocephalae (*Bai Zhu*), Pericarpium Citri Reticulatae (*Chen Pi*), Cortex Magnoliae Officinalis (*Hou Po*), and raw Radix Glycyrrhizae (*Sheng Gan Cao*). These were taken in the form of a decoction. Less than a year and (he) was at ease.

First, supplement the qi. Secondly, supplement the blood. Other medicinals (than these two kinds in my prescriptions) vary largely. But each case (I have attended) has been cured with their heaven-decreed life span preserved. Some may ask, "Qi (distention) (admits of) no supplementing method. How can your honor succeed in achieving recovery through supplementing qi? Is there really a theory that warrants your approach?" My reply is that it is the layman's assertion that qi (distention) admits of no supplementing method. In diseases caused by qi, (such as) glomus depression, congestion, and obstruction, it may seem hardly (possible to apply) supplementation for fear that it may worsen the disease condition. (But) what is not taken into consideration is that it is because the righteous qi is vacuous and no longer able to circulate and because the evil is stagnated and fixed and refuses to come out that the disease is produced (in the first place). The classic states: "Once sturdy, qi moves, effecting a cure; once dwindled, (qi) is fixed, producing disease." Suppose qi is dwindled but supplementation is not used, by what strength can it circulate?

Some may comment, "Your prescription is indeed carefully considered. But how slow it is in achieving an effect! Patients, long bed-stricken, must be tired of your roundabout way and pressing for a rapid (result)." My answer is that this kind of disease arose possibly three or five or even more than 10 years ago. Its root is deep and its condition is hideous. If one is anxious for a rapid effect, one is asking for a disaster.

(Only) those who know the kingly *dao*[63] are capable of treating this disease.

Some may ask, "Should one never prescribe disinhibitors at all in distention disease?" My answer is that if it is obviously known not to have arisen out of vacuity, if the disease (is) shallow, if the spleen and stomach are still robust, and if the accumulated stasis is not inveterate, and, in addition, if there are signs otherwise indicating precipitation, it is appropriate to administer coursing and abducting (medicinals) in a small way. (Some) may routinely take Zhang Zi-he's prescription, *Jun Chuan San* (Dredge the River Powder, or) *Yu Gong Wan* (Yu's Merit Pills)[64] to carry out a rapid attacking policy, (but I) really dare not.

---

[63] A kingly *dao*, as opposed to a tyrant's *dao* which denotes a high-handed or iron-fisted policy, mainly implies acquiring and maintaining rule with a peaceful and benign policy.

[64] This consists of Semen Pharbiditis (*Hei Qian Niu*), 4 *liang*, and stir-fried Fructus Foeniculi Vulgaris (*Hui Xiang*), 1 *liang*, which are made into pills with Succus Rhizomatis Recentis Zingiberis (*Sheng Jiang Zhi*). Da Yu was the famous legendary emperor who first introduced the slave system in Chinese history. He has been remembered over the tens of centuries for his successful harnessing of the Yellow River by means of dredging the river-bed instead of the then conventional way of building dams.

Treatise on *Shan Qi*[65]

Serious *shan qi* is an acute pain in the testicles extending to the lower abdomen. The pain may be in the testicles or in the neighborhood of point Five Pivots (*Wu Shu*, GB 27). In either case, it involves the foot *jue yin* channel. (*Shan qi*) may be tangible or intangible, silent or noisy. That which is tangible may be melon-shaped and that which is noisy may give a sound like a frog. Ever since the *Su Wen (Simple Questions)*, all the notable physicians in history have ascribed (this condition) to cold. Cold governs contraction and dragging. When exposed to cold, the channels and connecting vessels contract, leading to lack of movement (*i.e.,* lack of circulation of qi and blood and) thus causing pain. (Although) this is reasonable, there are cases of exposure to cold but without *shan*. (Therefore,) there must be another theory that can give a plausible explanation for this.

Once, I frequently had to walk on ice and wade in water because there was snow and ice plus knee-deep waters in front of my door. But I never became diseased with (*shan*) because I had never had internal heat in the past. This led (me) to think that this pattern (also) may originate from damp heat existing in the channels which has been depressed for an extremely long (time and is then) additionally bound by cold qi externally. (In this case,) damp heat evils have no way to disperse, thus giving pain. If (one) only posits (the

---

[65] *Shan qi* refers to swelling, pain, or insensitivity of external genitals, *i.e.,* specifically the testicles and scrotum.

85

existence of) cold, (the traditional theory) may well be imperfect.

Some may ask, "Since (only) the channel of the *jue yin* is (involved, which is) remote and located below, from where does (this) depressed, accumulated damp heat come?" My answer is that great taxation gives rise to fire in the sinews; intoxication and overeating give rise to fire in the stomach; chamber taxation gives rise to fire in the kidneys; (and) great anger gives rise to fire in the liver. When fire accumulates in an involved channel for a long time, the mother (channel) will generate (fire in) the child (channel), and, in case of vacuity, damp qi will become exuberant. The *jue yin* is ascribed to wood and is linked to the liver. (It) holds the office of general and is quick tempered. Because it is fiery and violent by nature, when bound by cold, it can be expected to give a great and fulminating pain.

My dull self (once) saw some (people) use Radix Aconiti (*Wu Tou*) and Fructus Gardeniae Jasminoidis (*Zhi Zi*) in equal amounts in the shape of a decoction and also achieve a rapid effect. Since then, I have never employed this formula as the basis (for my treatment of this condition), making certain additions and subtractions in accordance with signs and forms, but I have obtained a response. However, dampness and heat should be identified in respect of their quantities before treatment is accordingly carried out. Mere dampness (manifests as) much swollen *tui* disease.[66] There are also cases initiated by contained vacuity requiring the use of Radix Panacis Ginseng (*Ren Shen*) and Rhizoma Atractylodis Macrocephalae (*Bai Zhu*) with coursing and abducting medicinals as assistants. Upon examination, a pulse which is

---

[66] *Tui* disease refers to numb and insensitive swelling of the scrotum caused by cold and dampness.

found to be very deep and tight yet large and weak is the indicator (of dampness). In addition, the pain is moderate, (being) only a feeling of weight sagging and dragging.

Treatise on *Qin Gui Wan* (Gentiana & Cinnamon Pills)[67]

The cause of infertility is usually traced to the woman. Not seeking which parts must be responsible for the cause, (some) physicians find, in reading the ancient (compendia) of formulas, none other but *Qin Gui Wan* (Gentiana & Cinnamomum Pills) definite in (its) indications and specific in (its) designation (for this condition). Its composition of warm and hot medicinals seems quite humane. (These physicians thus) prescribe it with pleasure while (patients) take it with delight. Willingly, they bear the disaster of burning and parching, puzzled (at what has happened,) yet with no regret.

What is the matter? That which yang essence bestows, yin blood is able to contain. The essence forms the seed (or child)

---

[67] *Qin Gui Wan* consist of Radix Gentianae Macrophyllae (*Qin Jiao*), Cortex Cinnamomi (*Gui Xin*), Cortex Eucommiae Ulmoidis (*Du Zhong*), Radix Ledebouriellae Sesloidis (*Fang Feng*), and Cortex Magnoliae Officinalis (*Hou Po*), 3 *fen* for each of the above, processed Radix Praeparatus Aconiti Carmichaeli (*Fu Zi*), and Sclerotium Poriae Cocos (*Fu Ling*), each 1.5 *liang*, Radix Cynanchi Atrati (*Bai Wei*), blast-fried Rhizoma Zingiberis (*Pao Jiang*), Radix Achyranthis Bidentatae (*Niu Xi*), and Radix Glehniae Littoralis (*Sha Shen*), 1 *liang*, for each of the above, and Herba Cum Radice Asari Sieboldi (*Xi Xin*), 2.1 *liang*. Powder and make into pills with honey.

and the blood forms the wrapper (or womb). Thus pregnancy forms. Nowadays, infertility in women is largely due to blood being too scant to contain essence. There is, of course, more than one reason accounting for scant blood. However, if one desires to have a child, it is necessarily required to supplement yin blood. (This) must be made adequate before it is possible (to have a child). Since pregnancy presumes superabundant (blood), how reckless (those physicians) are when they use hot formulas which boil and simmer the viscera and bowels! If blood and qi are boiling, disaster will follow upon the heels (of such medication)!

Some may say that, if spring qi is warm and temperate, the ten thousand things generate and grow; (but) if winter qi is biting cold, all are killed and die out. Apart from *Qin Gui Wan* with their warmth and heat, what is able to make the child viscus (*i.e.*, the uterus) warm so as to form a fetus? My answer is that it is stated in the *Shi ([Classic of] Poetry)* that (when) harmonious and calm, a woman will be happy to have a child. At peace, qi and blood are not at odds. In quietude, yin and yang are not in conflict. (But,) having taken this medication, the channel blood (or menses) turns purplish black, gradually becoming decrepit and diminished, (and) the periods may possibly (become) early (or) possibly late. At the beginning, there may be a large food intake, but long after (*i.e.*, over time,) there arise a bitter taste and dryness in the mouth. (In that case,) yin and yang are not in equilibrium, and blood and qi are not in harmony. Diseases break out in swarms. How then is it possible to form a fetus? (And) even though a fetus is formed, the child to be borne is subject to disease and dies young. *Qin Gui Wan* consume and wear out the yin of the heavenly true. Be cautious and mindful!

Honorable Envoy Zheng's son, aged 16, asked for a treatment, saying, "Ever since (I was) seven months old, I have been suffering from strangury disease which launches a fit every five to seven days without fail. Whenever it attacks, there arises such a great pain that (I) slap the floor and call to heaven (for help). Only then does the water passageway move with about a cupful of a mixture voided something like lacquer and millet. After that, I can calm down."

I examined his pulse which was choppy when slight pressure was applied and wiry when heavy pressure was applied. Seeing that his form was thin and a little lanky and his complexion was green-blue and somber, (I) decided that his father must have taken great quantities of medicinals (prior to his son's conception) specific for the lower part and, in consequence, had left (this) heat in the fetus (with conception). This had (then) been retained in the child's life gate. Accordingly, (I) prescribed *Zi Xue* (Purple Snow)[68] which was to be mixed with finely powdered Cortex Phellodendri (*Huang Bai*), made into pills the size of Chinese parasol tree seeds, and thoroughly dried in the sun. Two hundred pills were administered in one dose, taken with hot boiled water only, and (then) pressed down with food. Half a day later, a fit of great pain appeared which involved (his) low back and abdomen. Then the water passageway moved with the voiding of a big bowlful of a mixture of something like lacquer and millet, and the disease reduced by eight of ten parts. Later Zhang Zi-zhong[69] prescribed him one *liang* of Pericarpium Citri Reticulatae (*Chen Pi*) and one half *liang* each

---

[68] This is known as *Zi Xue Dan* (Purple Snow Elixir) or *Zi Xue San* (Purple Snow Powder). It consists of gold (*Jin*), Gypsum (*Shi Gao*), Calcareous Spar (*Han Shui Shi*), Magnetitum (*Ci Shi*), Cornu Rhinoceroris (*Xi Jiao*), Cornu Antelopis Saigae Tartaricae (*Ling Yang Jiao*), Radix Scrophulariae Ningpoensis (*Xuan Shen*), Lignum Aquilariae Agallochae (*Chen Xiang*), Rhizoma Cimicifugae (*Sheng Ma*), Radix Saussureae Seu Vladimiriae (*Mu Xiang*), and Radix Glycyrrhizae (*Gan Cao*).

[69] Pupil and apprentice to the author

of Radix Platycodi Grandiflori (*Jie Geng*) and Caulis Akebiae Mutong (*Mu Tong*. These) were administered in one dose. Then about one *he* of the (same kind of) mixture was voided, and (the patient) was at ease. Since the father having received dry heat is capable of inflicting disease upon (his) child, what if the mother has received it? I am writing this with a view to corroborate the event of red-thread tumor (Li) Dong-yuan mentioned.

Treatise on Aversion to Cold Being Non-Cold Disease and Aversion to Heat Being Non-Heat Disease

The *Nei Jing* states: "Aversion to cold and shivering are both ascribed to heat." It also states:

Clenched (teeth) and quivering as if the spirit had lost its vigil are both ascribed to fire. Even though in a hot summer month, (if one has) aversion to cold, it is as if (one) is encountering wind and frost, and the body, even though covered with layers of cotton, may still feel chilly. Shivering and shuddering with clenched (teeth) are (descriptions of) the appearance of quaking and trembling. (Saying) the spirit is as if it has lost its vigil is (a way of describing) severe aversion to cold.

It is stated in the *Yuan Bing Shi (The Formulated Origins of Disease)*[70]: "If a disease (presents) severe heat (or fever) and, at the same time, contrarily there is a feeling of cold, this is actually a heat disease rather than a cold (disease)."

Some may ask: "Why is administration of hot medicinals often observed to achieve a little relief (in the case of this disease)?" My answer is that, in people with heat disease, their qi upflames and (becomes) depressed into phlegm-rheum. (This) inhibits and obstructs the clear path. (Since) the yin qi cannot ascend, the disease heat is particularly severe. When receiving heat, the accumulated phlegm may retreat temporarily. (However,) the force of the heat assists the evil, and the disease becomes deeper.

Some may ask, "Cold and heat being such, who dares to administer cold and cool (medicinals)! Are they not killing (if they dare to do so)?" My answer is that, when met with the pattern of shivering, the ancients might, in some cases, have achieved recuperation by employing *Da Cheng Qi Tang* (Major Support the Qi Decoction) to precipitate dry stools. Aversion to cold and shivering are obviously a heat pattern, but (this condition) should be (further) classified in terms of vacuity and repletion. The classic states: "Yin vacuity leads to the emission of heat." Yang, located in the external, is the defender of yin, while yin, located in the internal, is the guard of yang. If the essence spirit takes flight outward with inordinate lustful desire, yin qi is consumed and dissipated, while yang has nothing to which to attach. Therefore, it floats and dissipates in the muscular exterior, giving rise to aversion to heat. In fact, no heat exist, and (this condition) should be

---

[70] This refers to the *Su Wen Xuan Ji Yuan Bing Shi (The Formulated Origins of Disease Based on the Intricate Mechanisms of the Simple Questions)* in full, written by Liu He-jian.

treated as yin vacuity. It will be all right if (one) uses the methods of supplementation and nurturing.

Some may ask, "Aversion to cold is not a cold (pattern) and should be treated with cold medicinals, while aversion to heat is not a heat (pattern) and should be treated with supplementing medicinals. (This approach) is a shock to the ear and eye. Can you show us the (treatment) method clearly?" Below is my answer.

Advanced Scholar Zhou Ben-dao, aged over 30, contracted a disease of aversion to cold and asked me for a treatment when his condition became exacerbated after the administration of Radix Praeparatus Aconiti Carmichaeli (*Fu Zi*) for several days. I examined his pulse which was wiry and somewhat retarded and administered river tea with Succus Zingiberis (*Jiang Zhi*) and a small amount of sesame oil put in. (Subsequently, he) vomited about one *sheng* of phlegm. (His condition) abated by more than half. Zhou was very delighted, but I warned (him) that it was not yet time (for delight). Because there had been abundant dry heat and, moreover, (his) blood had been deeply damaged, it was necessary to take bland (flavored) food to nurture (his) stomach, and introversion was required to nurture (his) spirit. Only thus could water be generated and fire be downborne. Vigorously seeking promotion at that time, he was too fully engaged in social responsibilities to abide by (these) prohibitions and commandments. I observed that coolness and heat might be calmed to a small degree provided that blood-supplementing medicinals were administered in large amounts.[71] (However,) with lack of quiet both internally and

---

71 There is a very similar description of the same case given in Ch. 57, Bk. 4, of the *Dan Xi Zhi Fa Xin Yao (The Heart & Essence of Dan Xi's Methods of Treatment)* also published as part of Blue Poppy Press' Great

externally, kidney water would not be generated and latent toxins were sure to break out. After the disease was quieted (temporarily), he secured an appointment in Wu Cheng[72] requiring (him) to be on night patrol and (therefore,) to be affected by cold. (This) could be treated with nothing but Radix Praeparatus Aconiti Carmichaeli (*Fu Zi*). Because (he) was averse to raw Rhizoma Zingiberis (*Sheng Jiang*), sliced pig's kidneys had to be boiled with the Aconite. After three doses were administered, he was at ease. Knowing that latent toxins might easily break out (again), I advised (him) that he return home without delay. (However,) he thought (my advice) was (overly) fastidious. Half a year later, it turned out that (*ju*) broke out on (his) upper back and (he) died.

Again, Jurisdiction Administrator Shu had constantly felt heat in the feet below the ankles all his life. Even in winter he could not bear cotton-padded shoes. He used to say, "I boast a strong physique with no fear of cold." I told him that (the condition of) those feet indicated vacuity of the three yin (channels) and he had better break off sexual affairs soon so as to supplement and nurture yin blood. Thus (a disaster) might possibly be avoided. He smiled, giving no reply. Later at merely 50 years old, he was affected with atony and half a year later died. (One) can know the (correct) method of treatment from observing (these) two people.

Some may ask, "Is the disease of cold damage with aversion to cold and heat also a vacuity (pattern)?" My answer is that, in the case of diseases of cold damage, (evils) enter the

---

Masters Series, but there is a marked discrepancy concerning this sentence between these two places. The translator assumes that the *Xin Yao*, having been written later, is more credible.

[72] This is a county in Fujian Province.

internal from the external and the past sages have already given detailed discussions about this.

Treatise on Purplish or Black Menstrual Flow

Menstrual flow is yin blood. Yin must comply with yang. Therefore, (the menstrual flow) is red, assimilating the color of fire. Blood is the consort of qi. Thus it is hot when qi is hot and cold when qi is cold, ascends when qi ascends and descends when qi descends, congeals when qi congeals, stagnates when qi stagnates, is clear when qi is clear and is turbid when qi is turbid. Blood is often seen formed into clots which are (due to) congealed qi. Pain as the menses is about to move (*i.e.*, at the onset of the period, is due to) stagnated qi, while pain after menstruation is (due to) dual vacuity of qi and blood. Lightness in the color (of the blood) also indicates vacuity. (While) menstrual hemafecia with blood running frenetically is (due to) chaotic qi. A purplish color indicates heat in the qi, while black indicates severe heat in the qi.

If people point to wind cold indiscriminately whenever (they) see a purplish or black, painful, or clotty (menstrual flow) and (therefore) resort to warm and hot formulas, disaster will follow upon the heels (of such medication. This fallacy) can, in fact, be traced to the *Bing Yuan (Origins of Disease)*[73] which explains that the various menstrual diseases are all caused by invasion of cold wind. This, then, has come down unchallenged and become a popular (belief).

Some may ask, "Black is the color of the water of the north. Since purple is lighter than black, what is it if not (due to) cold?" My answer is that the classic states: "Hyperactivity never fails to do harm, (but it) can be brought under control when restrained." Severe heat invariably contains water transformation. Therefore, when hot, (the menstrual flow) becomes purplish, and when extremely hot, it becomes black. Besides, women are obstinate in nature and of base opinion with double sexual desire.[74] Therefore, inverted yang fire[75] in their viscera and bowels arises every day. What is this if not heat? If (this condition is due to) wind cold, it is invariably received from the outside. Even if there are such cases, however, they are but one or two out of a hundred or thousand.

---

[73] This is the abbreviated name of the *Zhu Bing Yuan Hou Lun (Treatise on the Origins & Symptoms of Disease)* written by Chao Yuan-fang (550-630 CE), president of the Imperial Medical Academy during the Sui dynasty. Chao was authorized by imperial decree to compile this book.

[74] In ancient China, women were forbidden to go outside their walled family compound. Confined to such a small environment with nothing to do but housekeeping and with no access to education, it is ironic that women in ancient China were believed to be narrow--minded by the men who kept them so.

[75] Inverted means counterflow or aberrant. Therefore, inverted yang fire refers to stirring ministerial fire.

Treatise on Gypsum

In terms of the names of the medicinals in the *Ben Cao (Materia Medica)*, although (the origins of) some are unknown, the majority are meaningful. Learners should not pass over these. Some are named for (their) color: for example, Radix Et Rhizoma (*Da Huang*, Great Yellow), Flos Carthami Tinctorii (*Hong Hua*, Red Flower), Radix Cynanchi Stauntonii (*Bai Qian*, White Front), Pulvis Levis Indigonis (*Qing Dai*, Cyan Black), and Fructus Pruni Mume (*Wu Mei*, Black Plum).

Some are named for (their) shape: for example, Radix Panacis Ginseng (*Ren Shen*, Human Homage), Rhizoma Cibotii Barometsis (*Gou Ji*, Dog Spine), Radix Aconiti (*Wu Tou*, Tortoise Head), Bulbus Fritillariae (*Bei Mu*, Pearl Shell), and Fructus Meliae Toosendanis (*Jin Ling Zi*, Golden Bell).

Some are named for (their) qi (*i.e.*, smell): for example, Radix Saussureae Seu Vladimiriae (*Mu Xiang*, Wood Fragrance), Lignum Aquilariae Agallochae (*Chen Xiang*, Deep Fragrance), Lignum Santali Albi (*Tan Xiang*, Sandal Fragrance), Secretio Moschi Moschiferi (*She Xiang*, Musk Fragrance), Fructus Foeniculi Vulgaris (*Hui Xiang*, Returning Fragrance).

Some are named for (some) property (of theirs): for example, Cortex Magnoliae Officinalis (*Hou Po*, Thick Simplicity), dry Rhizoma Zingiberis (*Gan Jiang*, Dry Ginger), Sclerotium Poriae Cocos (*Fu Ling*, Hidden Pollen), raw and processed Radix Rehmanniae (*Sheng Shu Di Huang*, Raw & Processed Rehmannia).

Some are named for (their) taste: for example, Radix Glycyr-rhizae (*Gan Cao*, Sweet Grass), Radix Sophorae Flavescentis (*Ku Shen*, Bitter Homage), Herba Lophatheri Gracilis (*Dan Zhu Ye*, Bland Bamboo Leaf), Radix Gentianae Scabrae (*Cao Long Dan*, Grass Dragon Gall), and vinegar (*Ku Jiu*, Bitter Wine).

Some are named for (their) ability: for example, Bulbus Lilii (*Bai He*, Hundred Convergence), Radix Angelicae Sinensis (*Dang Gui*, Expected to Return), Rhizoma Cimicifugae (*Sheng Ma*, Upbearing Flax), Radix Ledebouriellae Sesloidis (*Fang Feng*, Protector from Wind), and Talcum (*Hua Shi*, Lubricating Stone).

Some are named for (a period of) time: for example, Rhizoma Pinelliae Ternatae (*Ban Xia*, Midsummer), Herba Artemesiae Capillaris (*Yin Chen*, Based on the Previous), Semen Malvae Verticillatae (*Dong Kui*, Winter Malva), Gallus Domesticus (*Yin Ji*, Terrestrial Branch #3 Chicken), and Spica Prunellae Vulgaris (*Xia Ku Cao*, Summer Withering Grass).

Because Gypsum (*Shi Gao*, Stone Ointment) is (a substance) having undergone calcining in fire, grinding into powder, mixing with vinegar, and sealing in a cinnabar furnace, it is more solid and dense than tallow. If not capable of (being used as an) ointment, what use is it? It is named by both its property and ability, just as is Halloysitum Rubrum (*Shi Zhi*, Stone Tallow). Yan Xiao-zhong[76] assumed without reason that Calcitum (*Fang Jie Shi*) was Gypsum. Furthermore, Gypsum, sweet and acrid in flavor, is admittedly a medicinal for the *yang ming* which governs the muscles and flesh. Its sweetness can relax the spleen and boost the qi, quench thirst

---

[76] Yan Xiao-zhong was physician during the Northern Song dynasty and author of the *Xiao Er Fang Lun (Treatise on Formulas for Children)* published in 1119 CE.

and eliminate fire, and its acridity can relieve the muscles and promote perspiration. It goes up to the head and then enters the hand *tai yin* and hand *shao yang*. (Whereas,) in contradistinction, Calcitum is nothing but heavy in weight, hard in property, and cold in nature. If one tries to find ointment within it that is indicated for the three channels, where is that (ointment)? If a physician desires (the same) ability (from Calcitum as from Gypsum), this is equally difficult!

Treatise on Disease Necessarily Advancing in Case of a Large Pulse

The pulse (or vessels), which is the place where blood is, pertains to yin. Largeness, an equivalent to surging, is the display of fire (which) is ascribed to yang. In a disease caused by internal damage, yin is vacuous and overwhelmed by yang. Therefore the pulse is large. (This) should be treated as vacuity. In a disease caused by external damage, evils settle in the channels and the pulse is also large. (This) should be treated as overwhelming evil. (When) these two (conditions) are viewed together, the disease along with its signs in either case is just gaining momentum. Is it not appropriate to (thus) refer to the disease as advancing? (Wang) Hai-cang[77] calls

---

[77] Originally named Wang Hao-gu (1200—? CE), Wang Hai-cang was a noted physician of the Yuan dynasty and a prolific author of medical works, among which the most famous are the *Tang Ye Ben Cao (The Materia Medica of Decoctions)* and the *Ci Shi Nan Zhi (This Matter is Difficult to Know)*.

this "the sovereign encroaching on the minister." Whether his saying is correct or not, (I) shall be grateful to anyone who ever tells (me so).

An Analysis of Paragraphs and Sentences Concerning Disease Causes in the *Sheng Qi Tong Tian Lun* ("Treatise on the Communication of Life Qi with Heaven")

The *Li Ji (Records of Rites)* states, "The first (whole) year is spent in instructing how to break up the classics." This means that breaking down and analyzing the teachings in the classics consists of determining the ends of paragraphs and sentences. In the *Nei Jing*, there are four paragraphs concerning disease causes in the "Treatise on the Communication of Life Qi with Heaven." The first paragraph discusses cold as a cause. Counting from "it is desirable that it be like the movement of a pivot of the door," the three (following) sentences are irrelevant to the meaning of that which precedes (them. They) all (are left) dangling there. The two sentences, "The body is like burning charcoal..." and "When sweat exudes, it dissipates..." should be transferred to this place. When cold evils first lodge in the muscular exterior, evils will be depressed into heat. (This) is like burning charcoal and can be resolved with diaphoresis. This is (the

99

pattern for which Zhang) Zhong-jing's *Ma Huang Tang* (Ephedra Decoction)[78] is indicated.

The second paragraph discusses summerheat as a cause. Summerheat is a disease caused by sovereign fire. Fire governs stirring and dissipation. Therefore, there are spontaneous sweating, distressed thirst, and talkativeness.

The third paragraph discusses dampness as a cause. Dampness is the qi of earth turbidity. The head, which is the meeting place of the various yang (channels), is in a high position, and its body is vacuous (*i.e.*, hollow). Therefore intelligence and brightness is associated with it. If fumigated and steamed by turbid qi with (its) clear passages blocked, (the head) is heavy and dull as if shrouded or clouded by something. If timely treatment is lost, dampness is depressed into heat, and (this) heat may linger, refusing to leave. When the major sinews become flaccid and shortened, this is heat damaging the blood which is no longer able to nourish the sinews. As a result, hypertonicity arises. When the minor sinews become relaxed and lengthened, this is dampness damaging the sinews which are no longer able to bind the bones. As a result, atonic weakness arises. "Because of dampness" and "the head is as if wrapped up" each contain three characters (in Chinese) as a phrase. From "If damp heat is not eliminated..." down, each phrase contains four characters. The context is correct and the meaning is clear.

The fourth paragraph discusses qi as a cause of swelling, but no description of disease signs follows, there being probably omissions and lacunae. "The four linkings supersede each

---

[78] *Ma Huang Tang* consists of Radix Ephedrae (*Ma Huang*), Ramulus Cinnamomi (*Gui Zhi*), Radix Glycyrrhizae (*Gan Cao*), and Semen Pruni Armeniacae (*Xing Ren*).

other..." is irrelevant to that which precedes[79] it in meaning. (This is) also dangling writing.

Supreme Servant Wang[80] has said that the three diseases of summerheat, heat, and damp qi all can be thought of as started by the toxins of cold damage which progresses in order, producing diseases in a continuum. (He divided the above writing into) five sections which were taken as a single paragraph. I am skeptical about (this). Summerheat disease, if not treated, will lie latent to generate heat. Long-lasting heat will produce dampness. Long-lasting dampness will result in qi disease. Such cases are available. In the *Nei Jing* there is only (one such a statement that) damage inflicted by cold in winter, if causing no imminent disease, will give rise to heat disease in summer. (I) have never learned that cold toxins lie hidden and latent to start summerheat disease in summer.

As to damp disease, (the discussion) is a continuation of the preceding topic of heat. The head was said to be dampened contrarily (to its nature) as if wrapped by some wet article, wishing that the heat were eliminated. It is proper that "Because of dampness, the head..." be a sentence. (However,) if "as if wrapped by (something) damp" were made an (independent) phrase, then "the dampened head" and "wrapped by (something) damp" would both sound as if a

---

[79] Many scholars tend to interpret *si wei* as four limbs instead of four linkings which means four corners or directions. According to them, the sentence or paragraph as written by the author, "Because of qi, swelling arises, and *si wei* superseding each other, the yang qi is expiring", which can be found in the *Sheng Qi Tong Tian Lun* of the *Nei Jing*, should be understood as follows: "...swelling arises, and it appears in the four limbs in turn..."

[80] A.k.a. Wang Bing. See note 8, Zhu Dan-xi's Preface

performance of some person were involved. This would be incongruous with the meaning in context which is an enumeration of the diseases of cold, summerheat, (and so on). This does not allow for a lack of argument.

Some may ask, "The past sages spoke of warm dampness, cold dampness, and wind dampness, and (we) have never heard of so-called damp heat disease. (Even) when pouring over the *Nei Jing*, (one) cannot find it. Is your honor not lost in fastidiousness and vanity?" My answer is that, among (the diseases caused by) the six qi, those caused by damp heat make up eight to nine out of 10. The *Nei Jing* reveals damp heat. This is the first exposition (on the problem). The *Zhi Zhen Yao Da Lun* ("Great Treatise on What Is Consummately True & Essential") says, "If dampness ascends to an extreme extent and with heat...", and, in the text, it sometimes mentions dampness with heat existing in the center and sometimes heat with dampness existing in the center. This is a consummate and impeccable discussion of the *dao* (written out of) loving humanity by the sage. It is the Supreme Servant who was the first to make later generations in the world ignorant of the treatment of damp heat. If you would please return home for the *Yuan Bing Shi (Formulated Origins of Disease)* and give it a close study and detailed consideration, I would be grateful.

The Supreme Servant's Paragraphs and Sentences

In case of cold as the cause, it is desirable that it be like the movement of a pivot of the door. If daily life is as if (startled by) fright, the spirit and qi will float.

In case of summerheat as the cause, sweating and vexation give rise to distressed rapid dyspneic breathing, and stillness

102

gives rise to talkativeness. The body is like burning charcoal, and when sweat exits, (heat) will be dissipated.

In case of dampened head as the cause, (the head) is as if wrapped by (something) wet. If the heat is not eliminated, the major sinews become flaccid and shortened, and the minor sinews relaxed and lengthened. Flaccidity and shortening result in hypertonicity, while relaxation and lengthening result in atony.

In case of qi as the cause, swelling arises, etc.

Newly Determined Paragraphs and Sentences

In case of cold as the cause, the body is like burning charcoal. When sweat exits, (the evil) is dissipated.

In case of summerheat as the cause, sweating and vexation give rise to distressed rapid dyspneic breathing, and stillness gives rise to talkativeness.

In case of dampness, the head is as if wrapped up. If damp heat is not eliminated, the major sinews become flaccid and shortened, and the minor sinews relaxed and lengthened. Flaccidity and shortening result in hypertonicity, and relaxation and lengthening result in atony.

In case of qi as the cause, swelling arises, etc.

Treatise on Emptying the Granary

The classic says: "The intestines and stomach are a market." Although there is nothing they do not contain, they mostly contain grain. (Thus) they are called a granary (and) are like a barn for (storing) grains. Emptying means pouring out the old accumulation by flushing in order to make clean. The stomach which is located in the center is ascribed to earth. (It) likes to receive and hold but is unable to transport by itself. When people meet a mouth-pleasing kind of food and drink, it is not unlikely that they take in excess and are (consequently) damaged by accumulation. It is not unlikely (either) that partiality of the seven affects and thickness of the five flavors damage the virtues (*i.e.*, favorable qualities) of moderation and harmony. The remains of waste, retained phlegm, and static blood may become mixed and entangled together, accumulating with each passing day, and (get) deeper with each passing month. They are depressed and bound into gatherings and, when extreme, form something like the pulp of a walnut. (This produces) various kinds of odd-shaped worms (or parasites).

The central palace is no longer clear, and earth has lost the virtue of harmony. The inside being such, the external will (correspondingly) display either paralysis, consumption, *gu* distention, *lai* illness, or some unidentified, unusual disease. (For these,) the past sages designed *Wan Bing Wan* (All Disease Pills)[81] and *Wen Bai Wan* (Warm the White Pills)[82],

---

[81] *Wan Bing Wan* consist of Lacca Sinica Exiccata (*Gan Qi*), Radix Achyranthis Bidentatae (*Niu Xi*), and Succus Radicis Rehmanniae (*Sheng Di Huang Zhi*).

etc., resorting to a combined application of attacking and supplementation and to a compound use of cold and warm (medicinals) in the hope of hitting the disease conditions. (These methods) are indeed delicate and clever but not expedient or efficient compared with the granary emptying (method).

Buy 10-20 *jin* of bull's meat, choosing the fatter. Boil in river water till over-done (and) till it is melted in the broth. Filter out the dregs with a cloth to obtain a clear liquid, put (this) into the pot again, and simmer over a small fire till amber colored. Now it is finished. Drink a winecupful each time, continuing to drink at short intervals. A total of tens of cups should be taken in such a manner. In a cold month, (this) soup should be drunk warm. If the disease is in the upper, massive vomiting is desirable. If it is in the lower, massive diarrhea is desirable. If it is in the middle, both massive vomiting and massive diarrhea are desirable. All (this) is a flexible method in terms of (how) slow or fast (and how) much or little (to drink).

Beforehand, the patient should be arranged in a room which is bright and blocked (from drafts) in order to calm (him or her) down. Judging (by the amount of) that which is discharged, when the root of the disease has been exterminated, stop (the administration). Following the vomiting (and/or)

---

[82] *Wen Bai Wan* consist of Radix Aconiti (*Chuan Wu*), Radix Bupleuri (*Chai Hu*), Radix Platycodi Grandiflori (*Jie Geng*), Fructus Evodiae Rutecarpae (*Wu Zhu Yu*), Rhizoma Acori Graminei (*Shi Chang Pu*), Radix Asteris Tatarici (*Zi Wan*), Rhizoma Coptidis Chinensis (*Huang Lian*), blast-fried Rhizoma Zingiberis (*Pao Jiang*), Cortex Cinnamomi (*Rou Gui*), Sclerotium Poriae Cocos (*Fu Ling*), Fructus Zanthoxyli Bungeani (*Chuan Jiao*), Radix Panacis Ginseng (*Ren Shen*), Cortex Magnoliae Officinalis (*Hou Po*), Fructus Gleditschiae Sinensis (*Zao Jiao*), and Semen Crotonis (*Ba Dou*).

105

diarrhea, there may arise thirst, but it is not permitted to offer boiled water. The patient invariably will have long voidings of urine. Obtain and make (him or her) drink the urine which is called recycled wine. Administration of one to two bowls (of this) can not only quench thirst but flush away (any) remaining dirt (in the internal).

After one or two days of sleep, the patient will feel very hungry, and only then can (they) be fed some bland gruel. Not till three days after should they be given a little vegetable soup to nurture themselves. In half a month, the essence spirit will be felt invigorated, the formal body will be brisk and strong, and the inveterate infirmity will be overcome completely. Afterwards, it is necessary that beef be prohibited for five years.

My master, Xu Wen-yi, began with a disease of heart pain. He was administered dry and hot, sweet and acrid medicinals, such as Flos Caryophylli (*Ding Xiang*), Radix Praeparatus Aconiti Carmichaeli (*Fu Zi*), Cortex Cinnamomi (*Gui*), and Rhizoma Zingiberis (*Jiang*). As a result of more than 10 years of (such) treatment, his feet became severely hypertonic and painful. In addition, (he had) aversion to cold and copious retching. (Then) even Vermilion (*Ling Sha*), Galentitum (*Hei Xi*), Sulphur (*Huang Ya*), and Minium (*Sui Dan*, were administered), and (this was) followed by moxaing as many as over 10,000 cones. Various treatments were carried out for another several years and his pains became worse. He gave himself up as a disabled person, and the many (attending) practitioners were all at their wit's end. Another several years passed in such a way, when, because of distressed thirst and aversion to food for one month, he was administered *Tong Sheng San* (Communicate with the Divinity Powder) for half a month. (In consequence,) the great bowel (*i.e.*, the large intestine) was laid stress upon with rectal pressure and hot qi in the anus as if burning. Initially, what was evacuated was like motley-colored rotten silk and (then) like congealed Oleum Semenis Sapii Sebiferi (*Jiu Zhu Yu*). After half a month, the disease seemed to improve, and after another half month, a scant desire for grains appeared. But (still his) two feet were difficult to move with no one able to offer a scheme (of treatment). In the third month of the following year, this method (*i.e.*, granary emptying) was tried, and every step gained a response as indicated. Eventually he became a whole (*i.e.*, healthy) person. The next year, he had another male (heir), and 14 years after, (his) long life ended. Besides this, (I) have administered this medicine to a woman who suffered from years long foot qi. Vomiting and disinhibited (*i.e.*, loose) bowels were followed by ease.

Again, Xiao Bo-shan of Zhen Hai (county), Lord of a Myriad Households[83], personally tried (this method) for his urinary turbidity and uncontrollable (loss of) essence. (It) proved to be effective. (Yet) again, Lin, a friend (of mine) from Lin Hai, suffered from enduring cough with spitting of red (blood), fever, and emaciation. All (his attending) physicians considered (his condition) consumption, and none of a hundred formulas gained a response. I was sent for an inspection. The pulse was wiry and rapid on both hands. (His condition) was better by day and worse by night. No one had been able to offer a scheme (of treatment. He) also recovered thanks to this method. It was a winter month. The next year, he had a child.

Cattle are (ascribed to) *kun* earth, and yellow is the color of earth. (Cattle) have the virtue of *shun* (*i.e.*, going along [the correct way], or docility). The (curative) effect (of their meat)

---

83 This was a title of a commander in charge of an army in an area inhabited by roughly ten thousand households.

comes from their vigorousness, and the feat (of this meat) lies in making use of the male. Meat is a pleasure to the stomach. When cooked and reduced to a liquid, a shapeless thing, it dissipates headlong into the connecting vessels in the flesh. Via the stomach and intestines, it percolates and penetrates into the muscles, skin, hair pores, and nails, entering everywhere.

Over time, accumulations and gatherings will take a substantial shape, attaching to the thin turns and winding places of the stomach and intestines as their nests, obstructing humors and fluids, qi and blood, fuming and steaming, parching and burning so as to produce disease. Short of the miraculous intestine-scrubbing and bone-scraping, what is able to remove these? And how can a few spoonfuls or a few *zhu* (*i.e.*, 1/24 *liang*) or (even) *liang* of pills or powders (be expected to mount) a secret offence against the fence or wall, the door or window (of their nests)?

To the best of my knowledge, meat liquid tends to dissipate and seep. When the stomach and intestines receive it, they become twice as thick as before, seemingly swollen, and their thin turns and winding places are not as they were. The meat liquid brims, flowing like an inundating flood, and all the flotsam and old rotten substances are pushed, driven, and carried down with the current with no possibility of staying. That in the exterior turns into perspiration because of vomiting. That in the clear track spouts out with vomiting. That in the turbid track leaves with diarrhea. All the stasis and obstructions are washed away, and (everything) is settled. Beef integrates all the qualities of heaviness (*i.e.*, richness), freedom from impetuousness, and docility. (Beef liquid,) flushing and flowing, (is able to) moisten dryness and desiccation and to supplement and boost vacuity detriment.

108

How can it not afford the happiness of elevated and brightened essence spirit?

It is just like (the situation) after the Martial King conquered Shang. (At that time,) wealth was shared and millet was distributed to satisfy the anxious expectations of the Yin people.[84] This formula comes from a extraordinary person of the Western Regions.[85] After middle age, (normal) persons can (also) carry out (this granary emptying method) one or two times, and it can be an aid in preventing disease and nurturing long life.

Treatise on Ministerial Fire

The supreme ultimate (tai ji) engenders yang when it moves but yin when it is still. Yang moves and tends to change, while yin is still and tends to merge (with yang) so that water, fire, wood, metal, and earth are generated, each possessing one nature except for fire which possesses two. These are sovereign fire or human fire and ministerial fire or heavenly fire.

---

[84] The Martial King (Wu Wang) was the second king of the Zhou dynasty (11th century-256 BCE). The Shang dynasty (16th-11th century BCE) was the second dynasty in Chinese history, and its late periods were called Yin or Yin Shang.

[85] This refers to the areas west of Yumen Pass, including present-day Xingjiang and parts of Central Asia. This is a term left since the Han dynasty.

Fire with yin in the interior and yang in the exterior is that which governs stirring (or movement). Therefore, any movement is ascribed to fire. In terms of prestige, when (fire,) which is generated by form and qi, is fit in the five phases, it is known as the sovereign. In terms of position, (the fire) that is generated from vacuity and voidness keeps to its position to take orders. Therefore it is known as the ministerial (fire) which is visible because it moves. Heaven governs living things. Thus it is perpetually in movement. Once possessed of life, the human being, likewise, is in perpetual movement. The reason why (human beings) are perpetually in movement is none other than the work of ministerial fire.

That which appears in heaven and emerges from dragon thunder is the qi of wood. That which emerges from the sea is the qi of water. (The wood and water) that are present in human beings are accommodated in the two parts, the liver and the kidneys. The liver pertains to wood, while the kidneys pertain to water. The gallbladder is the bowel of the liver and the urinary bladder is the bowel of the kidneys. The pericardium is the consort of the kidneys. The triple burner is so named because it burns, with the lower burner in charge of the liver and kidney phase. Both (of these) are yin and (located) below. Without this kind of fire (*i.e.*, ministerial fire), heaven is unable to generate things. Without this kind of fire, human beings are not able to have life. Although coming from wood, the fire of heaven is always based on the earth. Therefore, if thunder is not hidden, the dragon not dormant, (and) the sea not fixed to the earth, they cannot boom, soar, or wave. Booming, soaring, and waving are (all) movements that produce fire. The yin of the liver and kidneys is in possession of ministerial fire which is common between humans and heaven.

Some may ask: "(If) ministerial fire is common between heaven and humans, then why did (Li) Dong-yuan believe it is the foe of original qi?" They may ask further: "Fire and the original qi are irreconcilable to each other. When one is victorious, the other must be the loser. Then what should be done so that neither of them is the winner or loser?" (My) answer is that Master Zhou[86] says that it is the spirit that illuminates consciousness, and when the five natures[87] are acted on by things, ten thousand matters come about. After acquisition of consciousness, the natures of the five, when acted on by things, cannot but stir or move. When speaking of movement, it means (the stirring of) the five fires[88] in the *Nei Jing*. Ministerial fire is easy to start, and, when the inverted yang fires[89] of the five natures fan each other, they stir frenetically. When fire breaks out from frenzy, its change is unpredictable, and it becomes existent all the time, boiling and simmering the true yin. Once yin is vacuous, there is disease, and once yin expires, there is death. The qi of sovereign fire is spoken of as summerheat and dampness in the classic, while the qi of ministerial fire is spoken of as fire in the classic. To demonstrate that it is more violent, impetu-

---

[86] This refers to Zhou Dun-yi (1017-1073 CE), philosopher in the Northern Song dynasty. Zhou was one of the founders of Neoconfucianism which was a combination of Daoist and Buddhist doctrines with Confucianism. These teachings had a profound influence on the academic circles of the Song, Jin, Yuan, and Ming dynasties.

[87] The five natures can be understood as the five organs or viscera of different natures or simply as the five viscera.

[88] *I.e.*, heart fire, liver fire, spleen fire, lung fire, and kidney fire

[89] Inverted means counterflow and yang is an epithet. Therefore, the term can be interpreted simply as counterflow of fire.

ous, vigorous, and fierce than sovereign fire, ministerial fire is said to be a foe to the original qi.

Master Zhou also says, "The sages stipulated (as norms) justice and uprightness, compassion and honesty, and advocated stillness." Master Zhu[90] says, "It is vital to have the heart of the *dao* be the governor of the whole body before the human heart obeys orders from it all the time." This is a good way to cope with fire. Thus, the human heart is put under the orders of the heart of the *dao* and is capable of being governed by stillness. (Then) the movement of all five fires will be under control. Ministerial fire can (then) do nothing but assist and supplement creation and transformation (and) can be used to perpetuate the generation of life. What kind of foe is there (then)?

Some may ask: "Ministerial fire in the *Nei Jing* is defined in the notes[91] as the *shao yin* and *shao yang*, and the *jue yin* and *tai yang* are never involved. (Therefore,) what is your honor referring to?" (My) answer is that once the foot *tai yang* and *shao yin* were mentioned by (Li) Dong-yuan. (Li) prescribed treatment (for these) with stir-fried Cortex Phellodendri (*Huang Bai*) based the consideration that its flavor is acrid (and) it is able to drain the fire within water. (Zhang) Dai-ren[92] also stated that, related to the gallbladder and triple burner, fire should be traced for the purpose of

---

[90] This refers to Zhu Xi, one of the seminal thinkers responsible for Neoconfucianism and one of the greatest Chinese philosophers of all time.

[91] This refers to the notes given by Wang Bing in his edition of the *Nei Jing*.

[92] A.k.a. Zhang Zi-he

treatment and that the case is the same with the liver and pericardium. All these refer to the fire of dragon thunder. I, too, have given a comprehensive explanation that both the heavenly and human fires are generated from movement. The discussion above is, in fact, an extension of the implications of (these) two masters.

Some may ask, "The Nei Jing speaks of fire in various ways which are usually met in (discussions of) the six qi but never in discussions of the viscera and bowels. Did the two masters (mentioned above) have other documentation? Could your honor point them out to us?" The classic states: "All the hundreds of diseases are generated from the movement and changing of wind, cold, summerheat, dampness, dryness, and fire." Qi Bo[93] enumerated nineteen disease mechanisms, among which there are five ascribed to fire. Does this not show that the ministerial fire that causes disease comes from the viscera and bowels? In reference to the Nei Jing, shao yang disease manifests with tuggings and slackenings. Tai yang disease (manifests with) occasional spinning collapse. Shao yang disease (manifests with) visual distortion, sudden loss of voice, oppression, and loss of consciousness of people. Are not the various kinds of heat with visual distortion and tuggings ascribed to fire? (In case of) shao yang disease with aversion to cold and shuddering and chattering, gallbladder disease of quivering with cold, shao yin disease with aversion to cold as after a soaking and shivering, and jue yin disease with aversion to cold as after a soaking and quivering with cold, are not the various kinds of clenched (teeth), shuddering and chattering as if the spirit's vigil were lost ascribed to fire? (In case of) shao yang disease with counterflow retching and ascension of inverted qi, urinary bladder disease with

---

[93] Qi Bo was the main teacher who dialogues with the Yellow Emperor in the Nei Jing.

upsurging headache, *tai yang* disease with inverted qi upsurging into the chest with (the qi in) the lower abdomen tugging the testicles and dragging the lumbar spine and upsurging into the heart, and *shao yin* disease with qi upsurging into the chest and counterflow retching, are not the various kinds of counterflow upsurging ascribed to fire? In case of *shao yang* disease with delirium and frenzy, *tai yang* disease with delirium and frenzy, and urinary bladder disease with mania and withdrawal, are not the various kinds of agitation and mania ascribed to fire? In the case of *shao yang* disease with dorsal swelling and susceptibility to fright and *shao yin* disease with visual distortion, fever with aching, and dorsal swelling with inability to stand for long, are not the various kinds of dorsal swelling, aching pain, fright and scare ascribed to fire?

In addition, the *Yuan Bing Shi (Formulated Origins of Disease)* states:

> The various kinds of wind shaking and dizziness which are ascribed to the liver are (due to) the stirring of fire. The various kinds of qi stuffiness and oppression and atonic disease which are ascribed to the lungs are (due to) the ascending of fire. The various kinds of dampness swelling and fullness which are ascribed to the spleen are (due to) the overwhelming of fire. (And) the various kinds of pain, itching, and sores which are ascribed to the heart are (due to) the maneuvering of fire.

All this (shows) that the fire that causes disease comes from the viscera and bowels. (Wang Bing's) notes, (however,) fail to bring (this) out. Chen Wu-ze[94] was well versed and

---

[94] A.k.a. Chen Yan of the Southern Song dynasty, known for his erudition and unusual talents, author of the *San Yin Fang (Three Causes Formulary)* or *San Yin Ji Yi Bing Zheng Fang Lun (Treatise on the Three*

intelligent, and he discussed sovereign fire as burning warmth and ministerial fire as the daily consumed fire. But (even) he did not go into detail. It is no wonder why in later generations there has been no lack of blind and deaf people. How regrettable!

Treatise on a Large Left (Pulse) Being Favorable for the Male & a Large Right (Pulse) Being Favorable for the Female

The lungs which govern qi have their pulse situated in the right *cun* section, and the spleen, stomach, life gate, and triple burner which change and function through the qi have (their pulses) next to it. The heart which governs blood has its pulse situated in the left *cun*, and the liver, gallbladder, kidneys, and urinary bladder which are tunnels and storehouses of essence blood have (their pulses) next to it. A male is conceived thanks to qi and is, therefore, governed by qi. A female is conceived thanks to contained blood and is, therefore, governed by blood. In a male with an enduring disease, if the right pulse is fuller than the left, there (still) exists stomach qi, and the disease, even though severe, is curable. In a female with an enduring disease, if the left pulse is fuller than the right, there (still) exists stomach qi, and the disease, even though severe, is curable. (Pulse images) contrary to this indicate severe vacuity.

Causes of Disease, Their Symptoms & Formulas) in full.

Some may argue, "(The pulses of) the heart, small intestine, liver, gallbladder, kidneys, and urinary bladder are on the left, while (the pulses of) the lungs, large intestine, spleen, stomach, life gate, and triple burner are on the right. The positions are the same for the male and female (alike) and are unchanging. The *Mai Fa Zan (The Method of the Pulse in Verse)* says, 'The left (pulse) being large is favorable for the male and the right (pulse) being large is favorable for the female.' In your explanation, not only are the right and left (sides) are reversed (in relation to the pulses), but fullness seems taken for largeness. Do you really have a theory to warrant your argument?" (My) answer is that largeness is, practically (speaking), a disease pulse (quality). Nowadays (when) largeness is taken as favorable, it has acquired the meaning of exuberance. Therefore, (I) am encouraged to use the word full (instead). The *Mai Jing (Pulse Classic)* is a work that tirelessly teaches physicians. (In it,) the left and right should certainly be spoken of in light of the (attending) physician. If the patient were taken as the rule, it would be a gross blunder, no less than a deviation of a thousand *li*!

Some may (continue to) argue, "In a previous passage (the *Mai Jing*) describes the liver and heart as emerging on the left and the spleen and lungs on the right with the left (pulse) governing (the diagnosis of) the viscera and the right (that of) the bowels. In a later part, the left is said to be *ren ying* and the right *qi kou*.[95] (Thus the left and right) are spoken of in light of the patient. How can (the text) be so self-contradictory?"

---

[95] Here, the terms *qi kou* (qi opening) and *ren ying* (human prognosis) refer to the right *cun* and left *cun* respectively of the radial pulse at the styloid process of the wrist.

The answer is that in chapter five, part nine of the *Mai Jing*, the beginning part provides a list of large, floating, rapid, stirring, long, slippery, deep, choppy, weak, wiry, short, and faint (pulses) which are mentioned in terms of yin and yang in regards to the images. In a later place, the expressions "in front of the barrier (*guan*)" and "behind the barrier" refer to a discussion of yin and yang (of the pulses) in light of positions. (As to) yin attaching to yang and yang attaching to yin, these are spoken of in terms of the yin and yang of blood and qi. All these are discussions about the yin and yang of the pulse, but they are inconsistent in (their) reference. (Such) a referential discrepancy in context does not justify doubt. The *(Mai Fa) Zan* says, "For a yin disease, treat the official (*i.e.*, the viscus). Does this not (mean) to treat the blood? "For a yang disease, treat the bowel." Does this not (mean) to treat the qi? Considering this, perhaps (my statements) do agree with the meaning of the classics.

Treatise on Eating Bland (Food)

Some may ask, "The *Nei Jing* states that insufficient essence should be supplemented with flavors. It is also stated that the earth feeds human beings with the five flavors. The ancients began to eat meat at the age of 50, but your honor, now as old as 70, (even yet) abstains completely from salt and vinegar. Have you acquired the *dao* (*i.e.*, achieved sainthood)? (If not,) how does your honor manage to keep your spirit thriving and your complexion shining?"

The answer is that some of the flavors are a gift from heaven and others are produced by human endeavor. The gifts from the heaven include, for instance, grains, beans, greens, and fruits which are moderate and harmonious flavors. When eaten as food by humans, these result in supplementing yin. These are what is referred to as flavor in the *Nei Jing*.

Those which human endeavor produces are the partially thick flavors made by means of brewing and blending in the process of cooking. These carry toxins that cause illnesses and fell life. It is these sort of flavors that you are suspicious of. Abstention from salt and vinegar is not truly eating bland. The saltiness in barley and chestnut, the sweetness in rice and yam, and the acridity in scallion and garlic, these are all flavors (too). Do you consider them bland?

The hearts of those who rest content with moderate and harmonious flavors are restrained and fire (in them) is downborne. Those who are happy (only) with partially thick flavors indulge (*i.e.*, let loose) overwhelming fire. There is no doubt (about this). The *Nei Jing* also states, "That which is generated by yin is rooted in the five flavors." These are certainly the flavors bestowed by heaven. And that which damages the five palaces of yin is (also) the five flavors. (But) these are certainly the flavors produced by human endeavor. Thus the teaching of the sage for the protection of the people is all-embracing.

People must eat whenever they are hungry. The virtue of earth is embodied in the sweetness and blandness of rice. Rice is a substance ascribed to yin and is most supplementing, but it should be taken together with vegetables. The reason why (it should be eaten) together with vegetable in order to replenish is the fear that it would (otherwise) cause detriment to the stomach if eaten in quantity when hungry or when excessively worried. Vegetables are taken to assist rice in replenishing and fulfilling because they are able to course and free (the stomach) and make transformation easy. This is the compassion heaven and earth cherish in generating things.

The *Lun Yu (The Analects)*[96] say, "However much meat (is eaten), it should not be allowed to overwhelm food qi." The *(Yi) Zhuan (Commentaries [on the {Classic of} Change])* says, "Though host and guest dine together all day long, pressing (one another) with a hundred prostrations, they should never drink more than three rounds in order to avoid a wine disaster." Here the sage hints (at the above) instructions. If fat and fish are taken with grain, their thick flavors enjoy the assistance of grain. (Therefore,) their accumulation will be long lasting. How can they not assist yin fire, resulting in toxins? Thus, if an elixir taker[97] abstains from grain, it is all right, but none of those who take elixirs and do not abstain from grain can escape from falling victim to their toxins. The *Nei Jing* says,

> Long (taking thick flavors) enhances qi. This is a law of substance transformation. And enhancement of qi over a long time becomes a cause for premature death. Those who are content with thick flavors do not think of this.

---

[96] The *Analects* are one of the so-called Four Books of Confucianism, the other three being the *Da Xue (Great Learning)*, the *Zhong Yong (Doctrine of the Mean)*, and the *Meng Zi (Mencius)*. The *Analects* are a collection of teachings of Confucius.

[97] Elixirs here refer to drugs made mostly from minerals and metals by alchemists in the hope of finding a panacea to free people from disease and prolong life. Such mineral and metals medicinals are hard to digest and tend to damage the stomach. Thus, if they are eaten with grains which tend to be somewhat difficult to disperse, the toxins inherent in these mineral medicinals will harm the stomach even more.

119

Some may ask again why insufficient essence is said to be supplemented with flavor rather than with qi. The answer is that flavor is yin, while qi is yang. To supplement essence with yin aims at the root. Therefore, those which supplement with flavor, for example, Radix Glycyrrhizae (*Gan Cao*), Rhizoma Atractylodis Macrocephalae (*Bai Zhu*), Radix Rehmanniae (*Di Huang*), Rhizoma Alismatis (*Ze Xie*), Fructus Schizandrae Chinensis (*Wu Wei Zi*), and Tuber Asparagi Cochinensis (*Tian Men Dong*), are all medicinals with thick flavors. When the classic states that vacuity is treated by supplementation, it means just this (kind of supplementation).

In a preceding passage, (the classic) states that insufficient form is treated by warming with qi. Damage from taxation fatigue causes qi vacuity, and, as a result, (the form) is insufficient. To warm is to nurture. Nurtured by warmth and conservation, qi is naturally replenished. Once qi is made wholesome, the form is wholesome. That is why warming is spoken of instead of supplementation. When the classic says that those who are taxed should be treated by warming, it means nothing but this. The compilers of the *Ju Fang* were ignorant of the resources of this (reference) and prescribed all sorts of warm and hot supplementing medicinals as assistants and aids for any vacuity detriment pattern, calling (their method) warm supplementation. They did not make (sufficient) effort to probe into the meaning of the classic.

Treatise on Counterflow Swallowing (*i.e.,* Hiccough)

Swallowing disease is due to qi counterflow. (In this case,) qi upsurges straight from below the navel and rushes out of the mouth making a noise. Thus (the disease) is so named. The *(Shang) Shu (Book of History)*[98] says, "Fire (tends to) flame upward." The *Nei Jing* says, "The various kinds of counterflow and upsurging are all ascribed to fire." (Li) Dong-yuan says, "Fire and the original qi are irreconcilable to each other." He adds, "Fire is the foe of qi."

Ancient formulas all regard (hiccough) as (due to) stomach weakness, never touching on fire. Moreover, they treat it with Flos Caryophylli (*Ding Xiang*), Calyx Diospyroris Kaki (*Shi Di*), Caulis Bambusae In Taeniis (*Zhu Ru*), Pericarpium Citri Reticulatae (*Chen Pi*), etc., without considering which can downbear fire and which supplement vacuity. The yin qi of human beings depends on the stomach for nourishment. When stomach earth is injured and reduced, wood qi bullies it. This is earth defeated by bandit wood. When seized by fire, yin is unable to hold in the interior, and wood carries ministerial fire with it to overwhelm (yin), surging directly upward along the clear passageway. When stomach weakness is spoken of, yin weakness is meant. This is a very severe vacuity. If this pattern is seen in a patient, it appears to be mortal. However, there may be (some complicating) repletion which should not be left unknown. (Let) me take the liberty to render an illustration of (this) issue.

---

[98] This is a book compiled by the disciples of Confucius.

Zhao Li-dao, aged nearly 50, was weak in physique and excessively angry. (One day) in the very hot seventh month, he was greatly hungry and asked for a meal, but his family failed to serve him immediately. So he flew into a rage. Two days later, he contracted the disease of dysentery. (Consequently,) he felt thirsty. He brewed himself cold water with honey. After drinking this, he felt very much relieved, and his dysentery also gradually got better. (Then all the troubles came again.) After five to seven days had passed in such a manner, I was sent for treatment. His pulse was a bit large but not rapid. Therefore, I told him to stop (drinking) the honey water. When thirsty, he was made to take a decoction of Radix Panacis Ginseng (*Ren Shen*) and Rhizoma Atractylodis Macrocephalae (*Bai Zhu*) brewed with *Yi Yuan San* (Boost the Origin Powder).[99] (His) dysentery gradually improved again. Seven or eight days later, he felt very tired with (counterflow) swallowing. Aware that yin was vacuous owing to protracted diarrhea, I bid him to continue with the above prescription. However, the dysentery remained to be stopped. In addition, he again drank diluted honey.

Three days passed with the (counterflow) swallowing not checked. People all grumbled that (my) prescription was not appropriate, proposing (he) drink (a decoction of) Rhizoma Zingiberis (*Jiang*) and Radix Praeparatus Aconiti Carmichaeli (*Fu Zi*). I told them that supplementing medicinals are not rapidly effective and that Aconite is not a medicinal to supplement yin. Administration of it was bound to lead to death. They asked whether (or not) taking much cool water soaked food would inflict cold. I explained that in such fierce summerheat, drinking cool (water) caused no cold and there should be no doubt about this. In due time, when the

---

[99]   A.k.a. *Liu Yi San* (Six to One Powder). This is comprised of six parts Talcum (*Hua Shi*) to one part Radix Glycyrrhizae (*Gan Cao*).

strength (of the medicinals) had built up, (the disease) would naturally be checked. Another four days later, (counterflow) swallowing stopped and (his) dysentery was also at ease.

Chen Ze-ren, aged nearly 70, a person who was used to a thick flavored (diet), suffered from an enduring disease of dyspnea which recurred and stopped irregularly. Early that autumn, he contracted dysentery with much reduced food intake. Five to seven days after (the contraction, counterflow) swallowing arose, and I was sent for an inspection. His pulses were all large and hollow. People all considered this to be hard to cure. I said that, in the case of a thin form, there was still something that could be done (for this condition. Therefore,) a decoction of Radix Panacis Ginseng (*Ren Shen*) and Rhizoma Atractylodis Macrocephalae (*Bai Zhu*) was to be taken with *Da Bu Wan* (Great Supplement Pills) to supplement blood. Seven days later and (the patient) was at ease. The above two persons (both) suffered from vacuity.

Again, a female was coming to the age to put up her hair. (She had) an impetuous temper and thick flavored (diet). In a summer month, she contracted (counterflow) swallowing as a result of great anger. Each hiccough made her whole body shake and rock with her spirit clouded and loss of consciousness of people. Inquiry revealed (that this was) a sudden disease. Seeing that her form and qi were both replete, (I) prescribed a decoction boiled from Rhizoma Panacis Ginseng (*Ren Shen Lu*). After a bowlful was drunk, several bowls of stubborn phlegm were vomited and a clouded sleep followed a profuse sweating. One day later, (she was) at ease.

Radix Panacis Ginseng (*Ren Shen*) enters the hand *tai yin* and supplements yin within yang. On the contrary, Rhizoma Panacis Ginseng (*Ren Shen Lu*) greatly drains the yang of the *tai yin*. In a female, fulminating anger makes qi ascend. The

123

liver governs anger, while the lungs govern qi. The classic says, "Anger leads to qi counterflow." When qi counterflows as a result of anger, liver wood takes advantage of fire to bully the lungs, and consequently, swallowing arises violently with clouding of the spirit. Rhizoma Panacis Ginseng tends to provoke vomiting. When phlegm is vomited completely and qi is borne downward, fire wanes and metal qi is restored to (its) position. (Thus) the stomach qi becomes harmonized and resolved.

Herba Ephedrae (*Ma Huang*) promotes perspiration, but its joints are capable of stopping sweat. Grain is ascribed to metal, while its chaff is hot in nature. Wheat is ascribed to yang, while its bran is cool in nature. (Our) Confucian predecessors stated that every substance is possessed of the supreme ultimate, (*i.e.,*) partakes of or includes both yin and yang. Students (are required to) gain (knowledge and understanding) by drawing parallels from inference and extending a meaning by analogy.

Treatise on (the Art of) Inside the Chamber Supplementation & Boosting

Some may ask, "In the *Qian Jin (Thousand [Pieces of] Gold)*, there is the art of supplementing and boosting inside the chamber.[100] Is it alright to use?" My response is that the *(Yi)*

---

[100]   The inside the chamber art or method refers to having sex but withholding ejaculation.

124

Zhuan states that happiness or misfortune, regret and shame are all produced from stirring (or movement). It follows that disease in human beings is also a product of stirring, and, in extreme, disease ends in death. To enable humans to live, the heart which is fire is located above and the kidneys which are water are located below. Water is able to ascend, while fire (is able) to descend. One ascends and the other descends continuously without an end and herein lies life's vitality.

The body of water tends to be still, while the body of fire tends to stir. Movement is easy but stillness is difficult. About this, the sages have not forgotten to give a word. Confucianists have established the teachings of putting the heart right, restraining the heart, and nurturing the heart. All this is for the purpose of preventing fire from stirring due to frenzy (*i.e.*, madness over personal desires). Physicians instruct (people) to keep unperturbed and indifferent (to fame or gain), to take (everything) as empty, and to hold the essence spirit in the interior. All this, too, is for the purpose of deterring fire from stirring due to frenzy. Ministerial fire is stored in the yin phase of the liver and kidneys. If sovereign fire does not stir frenetically, ministerial fire cannot but take orders and keep to its position. Thus, how can there be any malicious flame burning and scorching or wild force soaring and rushing (fire)?

In the *Yi (Jing), dui*[101] symbolizes a young maid and is (homonymous or rhymes with) *yue* which means pretty.

---

[101] This is one of the eight trigrams. It has a broken line above two solid lines. Each of the eight *gua* or trigrams corresponds systematically to a number of phenomena similar to the five phases. In terms of people, *dui* corresponds to a young lady.

125

When encountering a young man, (*i.e.,*) *gen*[102], it becomes *xian*[103] which means being affected without a heart.[104] (At this,) *gen* should come to a halt. The (supplementing and boosting) method in the chamber should be designed for *gen* to halt. If, (however,) *gen* is not made to halt, it cannot but turn into a bandit and robber. Then what kind of supplementation and boosting is there? According to my understanding of the implication of the *Qian Jin*, it is for those of robust age who are lustful and libidinous and whose water bodies are not so tranquil as before that the inside the chamber method is designed as an aid to supplementation and boosting. This (art) can be applied (only) in those sturdy in physique with a tranquil heart who can remain unstirred before an irresistible foe (*i.e.,* an attractive woman. This method) is not easy to perform for those without the heart of a sage or the bones of an immortal. The female follows the law of water, while the male of fire. Water is capable of restraining fire. One takes pleasure in booming, while the other takes pleasure in receiving. This is a natural law.

If the inside the chamber (method) were (commonly) used in order to supplement, many people would be killed. To make things worse, ever since ancient times, customs have become more and more sinful, and the physique and constitution (of the people) is becoming more and more flimsy. It is a hard job to interpret dreams to the muddle-headed.

---

[102] This is another of the eight trigrams corresponding to a young man. It is made from two broken lines surmounted by a single solid line.

[103] This is one of the sixty-four hexagrams. It is made from the hexagram *gen* (young male) below *dui* (young female). In this case, it represents intercourse between the male and female.

[104] The character *xian* is formed from *gan,* meaning to move or affect, without *xin,* the heart radical.

The Theory of Heavenly Qi
Pertaining to Metal

Master Shao[105] says:

> Heaven depends on earth and earth depends on heaven.
> (Thus) heaven and earth are mutually attached to each other.

The *Nei Jing* says, "(Earth) is held up by the great qi." Since the clear and turbid began to separate, heaven has been operating as qi in the external which contains water and earth has been lying in the center as the form which floats on water. This qi is what is called heaven. Because of its lack of extremity, (it) is called great qi. (It) is extremely clear, extremely unyielding, and extremely energetic. (Thus) it is ascribed to metal. If not extremely unyielding, it would be unable to contain water. If it were not extremely energetic, it would be unable to operate endlessly and to hold the weight of earth. If it were not extremely clear, its unyieldingness and energy could not grow and it could not be old since the time of antiquity.

Some may ask, "Although your ascription of heavenly qi to metal agrees with the symbolic implications of the diagrams in the *Yi (Jing)*, yet how can you directly speak of (great qi) pertaining to metal? Those good at the study of heaven must be able to produce evidence in terms of humans, (just as) those who are good at the description of greatness must

---

105   *I.e.,* Shao Yong (1011-1077 CE), eminent Neoconfucian philosopher of the Northern Song dynasty, famous for his expertise in the *Yi Jing*.

resort to a figure of speech of smallness. Will you please clarify (your approach) to me?"

The answer is that among all (living) things generated by heaven, humans are the most precious. That the figure of the human being simulates that of the heaven is borne out by a comparison. The lungs govern qi and correspond with the skin and hair in the external. The *Nei Jing* mentions yang as the external defender. Is not this just hair and skin? This is symbolic of heaven. The bones and flesh (and) viscera and bowels that are wrapped inside are symbolic of earth. Blood circulating endlessly day and night in the muscular interstices under the skin are symbolic of water. Taking a combined view of these three aspects, is it not valid to say that (as regards the human body,) water floats earth, heaven contains water, and earth is suspended in the center? When the sage who created the *Yi (Jing)* took metal as the symbol of qi, he did have justification.

Commentary Treatise on Zhang Zi-he's Attacking (Method)

My dull self has been reading Zhang Zi-he's books. They focus solely on the use of attacking. (This is based) on the point of view that the righteous qi is not able to cause itself disease. It is because of the invasion of evils that disease arises, and once (these) evils are removed, the righteous qi calms itself automatically. Illnesses may occur in the upper, middle, or lower, in the shallow or deep (part), and, according to (these) variations, diaphoresis, ejection, and precipitation are prescribed in order to attack (these evils).

128

At first sight of his books, one might conclude that all medical methods are encompassed in them. Later, I thought of the *Nei Jing* where vacuity is said to be the vacuity of the righteous qi and repletion is said to be the repletion of evil qi. Evils invariably invade because the righteous qi is vacuous. Thus, evil finds a chance to invade. If the righteous qi is replete, there is no possibility that evils can intrude by their own. With reference to this, (I) could not help becoming doubtful of Zi-he's methodology.

Further, (I) thought of the statements in the *Nei Jing* that say, "With yin calm and yang sound, the essence spirit is well governed; (but) with yin and yang separated, essence qi expires." I was also reminded of (Zhang) Zhong-jing who said, "If an illness requires diaphoresis for resolution and examination (reveals) a choppy pulse in the *chi* section, it is necessary to administer *Huang Qi Jian Zhong Tang* (Astragalus Build the Center Decoction) for the purpose of supplementation and then apply diaphoresis." On that account, I began to suspect that the works of Zi-he were not written by the brush (*i.e.*, the hand) of Zi-he. Well-known to middle earth, his (treatment) methodology must surpass that of his contemporaries. Then why does what is conveyed in his works differ so greatly from the implications of the *Nei Jing* and (Zhang) Zhong-jing? I was determined to find an illustrious master as a disciple who would open my stuffiness (*i.e.*, shed light on my confusion). Then I traveled mountains and waters, and, whenever hearing of someone practicing medicine somewhere, I would go to pay a visit and ask for instruction. I travelled several prefectures but found no one (worthy).

Not till when I was later in Ding Cheng[106] where I first had access to the *Yuan Bing Shi (Formulated Origins of Disease)* and

---

[106] This is the name of a county in present-day Zhejiang province.

the remedy books by (Li) Dong-yuan did I suddenly become thoroughly conscious of Zi-he's imprudence. However, I still did not get a well-founded teaching. I was saying that there was no one worth my while to learn from as a master in Jiang and Zhe[107] when, in the summer of the Yi Chou year during the reign of Tai Ding[108], I heard of Luo Tai-wu[109] and Chen Zhi-yan.[110] Then I set out to pay a visit (to Luo), only to be roundly rebuked five or seven times. (Thus,) I was put into a dilemma. I had lingered there for three months before I finally had the honor to be received. There I had a chance to watch Master Luo treating a sick Buddhist monk who had a yellow complexion (and) was thin, fatigued, and exhausted. Elder Born Luo examined his condition. (The monk) was from Shu.[111] He had left his mother at home when he set off to become a monk. He had been roaming in the Zhe region right to the river[112] for seven years when one day he suddenly was struck by the irresistible passion of

---

[107] This refers approximately to present day Jiangsu and Zhejiang provinces.

[108] The *yi chou* year was 1325 CE, and the reign of Tai Ding was from 1324-28 during the Yuan dynasty.

[109] Luo Tai-wu was a distinguished physician (?-1327 CE) who lived between the Song and Yuan dynasties. He is credited as the author of the *Tai Wu Xian Sheng Kou Shou San Fa (The Three Methods Orally Prescribed by Elder Born Tai Wu)*. In fact, this book was compiled by Zhu Zhen-heng, the author of the present work.

[110] We fail to find this person's identity. He was possibly a protegé of Luo Tai-wu.

[111] This is an ancient name for Sichuan province.

[112] In premodern China, the right was often referred to as the west. The river referred to is the Qian Tang River.

missing his mother. He intended to go home but (he) did not have the travelling expenses. From morning till night he looked into the West, sobbing in vain. Subsequently, he contracted the disease. At that time, the Buddhist monk was 25 years old.

Elder Born Luo had him lodged next door, every day entertaining him with beef, pig's tripe, sweets, and rich food, all of which were well done. More than half a month passed (in such a way). In addition, from time to time, he comforted the monk with consoling words. Elder Born Luo even (reassured him), saying, "I will give you ten *ding*[113] of money for you to make the trip home. I do not want you to pay (me) back but only wish to save your life from death." When he observed that the form (of the monk) had come back a little, he administered *Tao Ren Cheng Qi* (Persica Support the Qi [Decoction]) three times a day. (This) precipitating (formula) was not stopped till all (that was discharged) was blood clots and accumulated phlegm. The next day, the patient was fed only cooked vegetables and thin gruel. After half a month passed of maintenance and repose, the man became normal as before. More than another half month later, he was offered ten *ding* of money and started out. From this I greatly (*i.e.*, thoroughly) realized that the attacking method necessarily presupposes a person who is full and replete (and) sturdy in physique and constitution. Otherwise, when the evil is gone, the righteous qi is damaged. (Therefore,) a minor ailment will become a severe disease, and a severe disease will invariably end up in death.

Every day when patients came for treatment, Luo would first have the results of the pulse examinations reported. He used to just lie down listening to (these) reports. (Then, he would)

---

[113] This was the denomination of a metal coin in ancient times.

dictate a prescription of certain medicinals for a certain illness with a certain medicinal as the supervisor of those (other) medicinals and a certain medicinal as an usher into a certain channel. During a year and a half, there was not (one) set formula (prescribed). As to a particular prescription, it might be simultaneously attacking and supplementing, attacking first and supplementing second, or supplementing first and attacking second.

I further greatly realized that it is impossible that ancient formulas should agree with the treatment of present day diseases. This might be what is meant by prescribing to hit (disease) in accordance with the (changing) times. At (one) time, Luo also spoke of using ancient formulas to treat a present day disease, likening this to pulling down an old house to set up a new one. The wooden materials (of the old house) should be different (from those for the new one). Of what use are they if they have not passed the hands of the carpenter (and been reshaped)?

This reminds me of Master Xu who stated in his *Shi Wei (Expounding the Intricacies)*[114]:

> I read (Zhang) Zhong-jing's books and use Zhong-jing's methodology, but I never confine (myself) to Zhong-jing's formulas. Only thus can I claim possession of Zhong-jing's heart.

Later, I picked up the remedy books by (Li) Dong-yuan and hand-copied them. Consequently, I realized that the treatment of a patient ought to be like the lofty founder of Han

---

[114] This may refer to the *Shang Han Fa Wei Lun (Treatise Expounding the Intricacies of Damage by Cold)* written by Xu Shu-wei.

(*i.e.*, Han Gao-zhu, first emperor of the Han dynasty)[115] overturning cruel Qin[116] and the Martial King of Zhou overturning Shang. Following (their triumphs), if they had not distributed wealth and grain (to the people) and not stipulated the three rules of discipline[117], how could the damaged (national) qi and the fatigued and exhausted people have been reinstated? Therefore, I have decided that yin easily becomes exhausted, while yang easily becomes hyperactive, and (further,) that attacking (treatment) requires particular prudence, protecting the righteous qi by all means. A lesson should be learned from the *Ju Fang*!

---

[115] A.k.a. Liu Bang (256-195 BCE), the first emperor of Han dynasty (206 BCE-220 CE)

[116] *I.e.*, the Qin dynasty (221-207 BCE)

[117] During the wars against Qin, Liu Bang set up very strict disciplines for his armies preventing his soldiers from burning, raping, robbing, and looting. The contents of the famous three rules of discipline mainly concern the protection of the people.

Index

A

lower abdomen, qi mass in the middle of 45
agitation and mania 114
An Annotated Treatise on Cold Damage 76
ascension of inverted qi 113
atonic inversion 14
atonic weakness 100

B

Bend Middle 37, 41
bian zheng lun zhi methodology xi
Bing Yuan 57, 95
Bl 40 37, 41
blood, blackish 38, 46
blood clots, blackish 46
blood entering the channels and connecting vessels, malign 37
Board's Formulary ix
body heat 7, 31
Book of History 121
bowels, loose 11, 33
breast-feeding mothers 62
breasts, hardness of the 62
breast rock, suckling 64
Bu Tu Pai xi

C

chamber taxation 79, 86
Chao Yuan-fang 57, 95
Chen Liang-fu 59
Chen Shi-wen ix
Chen Wu-ze 114
Chen Yan 114
Chen Ze-ren 123
Chen Zi-ming 59
Cheng Qi Tang 44, 69, 91

Cheng Wu-ji 76
chest, qi upsurging into 114
child's palace 65
Chu Cheng 64-65
Chu Shi Yi Shu 64-65
Chun Xuan Wan 68-69
Ci Shi Nan Zhi 98
Classic of Change 3
Classic of Rites 71
clots, pepper seed-like 46
cold, aversion to 44, 90-93, 106, 113
cold without exposure to wind 15
Complete Collection of Fine Formulas for Women 59
complexion, purplish 45
Confucian scholar (physicians) 17
Confucius 119, 121
Corrected & Collected Formulas of the Great Harmony Imperial Grace ix
counterflow retching 113-114

D

Da Bu Wan 123
Da Cheng Qi Tang 91
Da Da Sheng San 59
Da Shun San 28
Da Xue 119
Da Yu 84
Dan Xi Zhi Fa Xin Yao vii, 93
Dang Gui Long Hui Wan 11
dao vii, ix, xii, 1, 3, 15, 20, 22, 47, 65, 84, 92, 102, 112, 117, 122
dao, heart of the 112
dao, kingly 84
dao, medical ix
delirium and frenzy 114
delivery, difficult 58, 60
diaphragm, oppression at the 9
diarrhea 9, 10, 23, 31, 34, 44, 68, 105, 106, 108, 122

OTHER BOOKS ON CHINESE MEDICINE
AVAILABLE FROM BLUE POPPY PRESS

3450 Penrose Place, Suite 110, Boulder, CO 80301
For ordering 1-800-487-9296 PH. 303\447-8372 FAX 303\245-8362
Email: bpeinc1@cs.com Website: www.bluepoppy.com

**A NEW AMERICAN ACUPUNC-
TURE** by Mark Seem, ISBN 0-936185-44-9

**ACUPOINT POCKET
REFERENCE** ISBN 0-936185-93-7

**ACUPUNCTURE AND MOXI-
BUSTION FORMULAS &
TREATMENTS** by Cheng Dan-an, trans.
by Wu Ming, ISBN 0-936185-68-6

**ACUPUNCTURE PHYSICAL
MEDICINE: An Acupuncture
Touchpoint Approach to the Treatment of
Chronic Pain, Fatigue, and Stress Disorders**
by Mark Seem ISBN 1-891845-13-6

**ACUTE ABDOMINAL SYN-
DROMES: Diagnosis & Treatment
by Combined Chinese-Western
Med.** by Alon Marcus, ISBN 0-936185-31-7

**AGING & BLOOD STASIS: A
New Approach to TCM Geriatrics**
by Yan De-xin, ISBN 0-936185-63-5

**AIDS & ITS TREATMENT
ACCORDING TO TRADI-
TIONAL CHINESE MEDICINE** by
Huang Bing-shan, trans. by Fu-Di & Bob
Flaws, ISBN 0-936185-28-7

**BETTER BREAST HEALTH
NATURALLY with CHINESE
MEDICINE** by Honora Lee Wolfe & Bob
Flaws ISBN 0-936185-90-2

**THE BOOK OF JOOK: Chinese
Medicinal Porridges, An
Alternative to the Typical Western
Breakfast** by B. Flaws, ISBN0-936185-60-0

**CHINESE MEDICAL PALMIS-
TRY: Your Health in Your Hand** by
Zong Xiao-fan & Gary Liscum, ISBN 0-936185-
64-3

**CHINESE MEDICINAL TEAS:
Simple, Proven, Folk Formulas for
Common Diseases & Promoting
Health** by Zong Xiao-fan & Gary Liscum,
ISBN 0-936185-76-7

**CHINESE MEDICINAL WINES &
ELIXIRS** Bob Flaws, ISBN 0-936185-58-9

**CHINESE PEDIATRIC MASSAGE
THERAPY: A Parent's & Practi-
tioner's Guide to the Prevention &
Treatment of Childhood Illness** by Fan
Ya-li, ISBN 0-936185-54-6

**CHINESE SELF-MASSAGE
THERAPY: The Easy Way to
Health** by Fan Ya-li ISBN 0-936185-74-0

**THE CLASSIC OF DIFFI-
CULTIES: A Translation of the *Nan
Jing*** ISBN 1-891845-07-1

**A COMPENDIUM OF TCM PAT-
TERNS & TREATMENTS** by Bob
Flaws & Daniel Finney, ISBN 0-936185-70-8

**CURING ARTHRITIS
NATURALLY WITH CHINESE
MEDICINE** by Douglas Frank & Bob Flaws
ISBN 0-936185-87-2

**CURING DEPRESSION
NATURALLY WITH CHINESE
MEDICINE** by Rosa Schnyer & Bob Flaws
ISBN 0-936185-94-5

THE HEART TRANSMISSION OF MEDICINE by Liu Yi-ren, trans. by Yang Shou-zhong ISBN 0-936185-83-X

HIGHLIGHTS OF ANCIENT ACUPUNCTURE PRESCRIPTIONS trans. by Wolfe & Crescenz ISBN 0-936185-23-6

HOW TO WRITE A TCM HERBAL FORMULA: A Logical Methodology for the Formulation & Administration of Chinese Herbal Medicine in Decoction by Bob Flaws, ISBN 0-936185-49-X

IMPERIAL SECRETS OF HEALTH & LONGEVITY by Bob Flaws, ISBN 0-936185-51-1

KEEPING YOUR CHILD HEALTHY WITH CHINESE MEDICINE by Bob Flaws, ISBN 0-936185-71-6

THE LAKESIDE MASTER'S STUDY OF THE PULSE by Li Shi-zhen, trans. by Bob Flaws, ISBN 1-891845-01-2

Li Dong-yuan's TREATISE ON THE SPLEEN & STOMACH, *A Translation of the Pi Wei Lun* by Yang & Li, ISBN 0-936185-41-4

LOW BACK PAIN: Care & Prevention with Chinese Medicine by Douglas Frank, ISBN 0-936185-66-X

MASTER HUA'S CLASSIC OF THE CENTRAL VISCERA by Hua Tuo, ISBN 0-936185-43-0

MASTER TONG'S ACUPUNCTURE: An Ancient Alternative Style in Modern Clinical Practice by Miriam Lee 0-926185-37-6

THE MEDICAL I CHING: Oracle of the Healer Within by Miki Shima, OMD, ISBN 0-936185-38-4

MANAGING MENOPAUSE NATURALLY with Chinese Medicine by Honora Wolfe ISBN 0-936185-98-8

PAO ZHI: Introduction to Processing Chinese Medicinals to Enhance Their Therapeutic Effect, by Philippe Sionneau, ISBN 0-936185-62-1

PATH OF PREGNANCY, VOL. I, Gestational Disorders by Bob Flaws, ISBN 0-936185-39-2

PATH OF PREGNANCY, Vol. II, Postpartum Diseases by Bob Flaws. ISBN 0-936185-42-2

PEDIATRIC BRONCHITIS: Its Cause, Diagnosis & Treatment According to TCM trans. by Gao Yu-li and Bob Flaws, ISBN 0-936185-26-0

PRINCE WEN HUI'S COOK: Chinese Dietary Therapy by Bob Flaws & Honora Lee Wolfe, ISBN 0-912111-05-4, $12.95 (Published by Paradigm Press)

THE PULSE CLASSIC: A Translation of the *Mai Jing* by Wang Shu-he, trans. by Yang Shou-zhong ISBN 0-936185-75-9

THE SECRET OF CHINESE PULSE DIAGNOSIS by Bob Flaws, ISBN 0-936185-67-8

SEVENTY ESSENTIAL TCM FORMULAS FOR BEGINNERS by Bob Flaws, ISBN 0-936185-59-7

SHAOLIN SECRET FORMULAS for Treatment of External Injuries, by De Chan, ISBN 0-936185-08-2

STATEMENTS OF FACT IN TRADITIONAL CHINESE MEDICINE by Bob Flaws, ISBN 0-936185-52-X